This Book Belongs To:

_____

If Found Call:

_____

Published by:
Aromatic Publishing
Selinsgrove, PA

My Book of Blends / Liz Fulcher & Natalie Marie Collins - 1st ed.
ISBN-13: 978-0692587157
ISBN-10: 0692587152

Cover and Interior Designed by:
Natalie Marie Collins - NatalieMarieCollins.com

my BOOK *of* BLENDS

Where I keep all my favorite
essential oil and hydrosol
blend recipes safe

Dedication

For those who are helping the world heal
through the power of essential oils and hydrosols.

We thank you.

With Much Love,

Liz & Natalie

Meet The Authors

Liz Fulcher

Liz brings 24 years of experience as a Clinical Aromatherapist and Essential Oil Educator and offers both in-person and online classes. She is the Pennsylvania Director for the National Association for Holistic Aromatherapy (naha.org). Liz offers an acclaimed 235-hour Aromatherapy Certification Program.
Her website is: AromaticWisdomInstitute.com

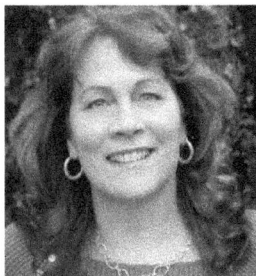

Natalie Marie Collins

Natalie is a healthy business coach & essential oil enthusiast as well as a Young Living Independent Distributor (#2734993) who helps others transform their businesses and lives into happiness through practical planning, easy action steps and balanced, healthy living.
You can find her at: NatalieMarieCollins.com

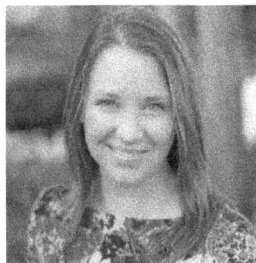

Carriers

If you are just getting started with essential oils, it can be overwhelming and confusing to understand how to make blends, what carrier to use and how many drops to add to those carriers.

Essential oils are highly concentrated plant extracts and some may be irritating to the skin if not blended in a carrier. When using essential oils topically, it's important to mix them into a vegetable-based oil or unscented cream to avoid skin irritation or sensitization. Use Organic when possible.

Using a carrier oil or cream ensures you stay safe.

Here is a list of commonly used carriers that are not only safe, but also nourishing to the skin and add a lovely healing element to your blends *:

Almond oil
Aloe vera gel
Apricot kernel oil
Avocado oil
Calendula oil
Evening primrose oil
Grape seed oil
Hazelnut oil
Jojoba oil
Macadamia oil
Olive oil
Pumpkin seed oil
Rosehip oil
Safflower oil
Sesame oil
Sunflower oil
Unscented lotion/cream
Walnut oil
Wheatgerm oil

*NOTE: If you have a known allergy or sensitivity to one of the above carriers, please avoid in the event of an allergic reaction. If you are unsure about your sensitivity to a carrier, try a small amount on the inside of your elbow to test for a possible reaction.

If you are unsure about your sensitivity to it, try a very small amount of the oil on a small patch of your skin to test for any reactions prior to making and using any blends with it.

Blending Guidelines

Here are some simple but important guidelines to follow to ensure you make safe and effective blends to use on the skin:

Weight of Carrier	1% Dilution	2% Dilution	3% Dilution
1 oz carrier	5-6 drops	10-12 drops	15-18 drops
2 oz carrier	10-12 drops	20-24 drops	30-36 drops

1% Dilution: This dilution is used for children under 12, and seniors over 65, pregnant women and people with long-term illnesses or immune systems disorders. A 1% dilution is also a good place to start with individuals who are generally sensitive to fragrances, chemicals or other environmental pollutants.

2% Dilution: This dilution is used on adults in good health for blends that support skin care, for natural perfumes, bath oils, and blends you use everyday or long-term.

3% Dilution: This dilution is used when creating a blend for an acute injury, pain relief or getting through a cold or flu. Blends made at this dilution are used only for a week or two.

Neat: Using essential oils "neat" (meaning undiluted – essential oil without any carrier) is inadvisable except in very specific situations. There are two reasons for this: 1) you can develop a sensitivity to the oils; and 2) many essential oils are too irritating to use without dilution. Oils can be used neat as follows: Small specific areas, acute situations (cut or wound, bee sting, bug bite and burn) and for short-term use. These must be highest quality, non-oxidized oils.

How To Use This Book
(from left to right)

My Blends Index: Write down your blend titles on the blank index lines so you can easily find and organize your blends.

Love Factor: This is your own personal rating system on how much you love the blend you created.

Blend Names: Every blend needs a name. This is fun, make it personal and you'll have an easier time remembering its purpose later.

How To Use: There are 3 main ways to use essential oils and hydrosols. Topically, through Inhalation and Internally. You will want to note how the blend is intended to be used.

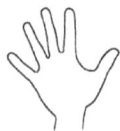

Hand = Topically

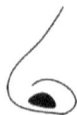

Nose = Inhalation

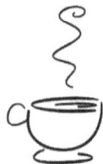

Cup = Internally*

*See Safety Note on page 13

Purpose: Note the purpose for this blend, what it helps to heal/enhance, who you made it for and why.

Ingredients: Be sure to note what essential oil(s) and/or hydrosol(s) you used and how many drops, along with the carrier oil(s) used (if any) in your blend so you can make it again and again - and so can your friends!

Notes: Write down any notes or things you noticed while making that particular blend or want to remember about it later.

Preparation: Write down your step-by-step instructions on how you prepared your blend.

Safety Note

*It is not recommended to take essential oils internally unless you know they are from a reliable source, are high grade and you have ample knowlege on which oils and the amounts that are safe to use. Essential oils work best externally.

Since Hydrosols are water based, they are safe to take internally.

My Blends Index

Blend Name	Page #

Blend Name	Page #

Blend Name   Page #

_____   _____
_____   _____
_____   _____
_____   _____
_____   _____
_____   _____
_____   _____
_____   _____
_____   _____
_____   _____
_____   _____
_____   _____
_____   _____
_____   _____
_____   _____
_____   _____
_____   _____
_____   _____
_____   _____
_____   _____
_____   _____
_____   _____
_____   _____
_____   _____
_____   _____
_____   _____
_____   _____
_____   _____
_____   _____
_____   _____
_____   _____

Blend Name	Page #

Blend Name   Page #

_____   _____
_____   _____
_____   _____
_____   _____
_____   _____
_____   _____
_____   _____
_____   _____
_____   _____
_____   _____
_____   _____
_____   _____
_____   _____
_____   _____
_____   _____
_____   _____
_____   _____
_____   _____
_____   _____
_____   _____
_____   _____
_____   _____
_____   _____
_____   _____
_____   _____
_____   _____
_____   _____
_____   _____
_____   _____
_____   _____
_____   _____
_____   _____
_____   _____

Blend Name	Page #

My Blends

Blend Name

Love Factor
♡♡♡♡♡
How To Use

Ingredients ◊

Essential Oil (EO) and/or Hydrosol (H) Used _____

EO/H _____ # of drops _____ _____
EO/H _____ # of drops _____ _____
EO/H _____ # of drops _____ _____
EO/H _____ # of drops _____ _____
EO/H _____ # of drops _____ _____
EO/H _____ # of drops _____ _____

Purpose

_____

Carrier Oils (CO) Used

CO _____ amount_____ _____
CO _____ amount_____ _____
CO _____ amount_____ _____

Preparation

_____
_____
_____
_____
_____
_____
_____
_____
_____
_____
_____
_____
_____
_____
_____
_____

Notes ✏

_____
_____
_____
_____
_____
_____
_____
_____
_____
_____
_____
_____
_____
_____

23

Love Factor

♡ ♡ ♡ ♡ ♡

How To Use

Blend Name

Purpose

_____
_____
_____
_____
_____
_____
_____
_____
_____
_____
_____

Ingredients

Essential Oil (EO) and/or Hydrosol (H) Used

EO/H _____ # of drops _____
EO/H _____ # of drops _____
EO/H _____ # of drops _____
EO/H _____ # of drops _____
EO/H _____ # of drops _____
EO/H _____ # of drops _____

Carrier Oils (CO) Used

CO _____ amount_____
CO _____ amount_____
CO _____ amount_____

Notes

_____
_____
_____
_____
_____
_____
_____
_____
_____
_____
_____
_____
_____
_____

Preparation

_____
_____
_____
_____
_____
_____
_____
_____
_____
_____
_____
_____
_____
_____
_____
_____
_____

Blend Name

Love Factor
♡ ♡ ♡ ♡ ♡

How To Use

Ingredients 💧

Essential Oil (EO) and/or Hydrosol (H) Used

EO/H _____ # of drops _____

EO/H _____ # of drops _____

EO/H _____ # of drops _____

EO/H _____ # of drops _____

EO/H _____ # of drops _____

EO/H _____ # of drops _____

Carrier Oils (CO) Used

CO _____ amount_____

CO _____ amount_____

CO _____ amount_____

Preparation

_____

_____

_____

_____

_____

_____

_____

_____

_____

_____

_____

_____

_____

_____

_____

_____

Purpose

_____

_____

_____

_____

_____

_____

_____

_____

_____

_____

_____

Notes ✏️

_____

_____

_____

_____

_____

_____

_____

_____

_____

_____

_____

_____

_____

_____

Love Factor

♡ ♡ ♡ ♡ ♡

How To Use

Blend Name

Purpose

_____
_____
_____
_____
_____
_____
_____
_____
_____
_____
_____
_____

Ingredients ◊

Essential Oil (EO) and/or **Hydrosol (H) Used**

EO/H _____ # of drops _____
EO/H _____ # of drops _____
EO/H _____ # of drops _____
EO/H _____ # of drops _____
EO/H _____ # of drops _____
EO/H _____ # of drops _____

Carrier Oils (CO) Used

CO _____ amount_____
CO _____ amount_____
CO _____ amount_____

Notes ✏

_____
_____
_____
_____
_____
_____
_____
_____
_____
_____
_____
_____
_____
_____

Preparation

_____
_____
_____
_____
_____
_____
_____
_____
_____
_____
_____
_____
_____
_____
_____
_____
_____

Blend Name

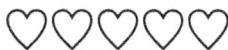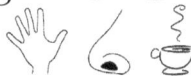

Ingredients ⬡

Purpose

Essential Oil (EO) and/or Hydrosol (H) Used _____

EO/H _____ # of drops _____ _____
EO/H _____ # of drops _____ _____
EO/H _____ # of drops _____ _____
EO/H _____ # of drops _____ _____
EO/H _____ # of drops _____ _____
EO/H _____ # of drops _____ _____

_____

Carrier Oils (CO) Used

_____
CO _____ amount_____ _____
CO _____ amount_____ _____
CO _____ amount_____ _____

Preparation

Notes ✏

_____ _____
_____ _____
_____ _____
_____ _____
_____ _____
_____ _____
_____ _____
_____ _____
_____ _____
_____ _____
_____ _____
_____ _____
_____ _____
_____ _____
_____ _____
_____ _____
_____ _____
_____ _____

27

Love Factor

♡ ♡ ♡ ♡ ♡

How To Use

Blend Name

Purpose

_____
_____
_____
_____
_____
_____
_____
_____
_____
_____
_____

Ingredients

Essential Oil (EO) and/or Hydrosol (H) Used

EO/H _____ # of drops _____
EO/H _____ # of drops _____
EO/H _____ # of drops _____
EO/H _____ # of drops _____
EO/H _____ # of drops _____
EO/H _____ # of drops _____

Carrier Oils (CO) Used

CO _____ amount_____
CO _____ amount_____
CO _____ amount_____

Notes

_____
_____
_____
_____
_____
_____
_____
_____
_____
_____
_____
_____
_____

Preparation

_____
_____
_____
_____
_____
_____
_____
_____
_____
_____
_____
_____
_____
_____

Blend Name

Love Factor
♡♡♡♡♡

How To Use
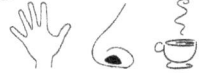

Ingredients 🜄

Essential Oil (EO) and/or Hydrosol (H) Used

EO/H _____ # of drops _____

EO/H _____ # of drops _____

EO/H _____ # of drops _____

EO/H _____ # of drops _____

EO/H _____ # of drops _____

EO/H _____ # of drops _____

Carrier Oils (CO) Used

CO _____ amount_____

CO _____ amount_____

CO _____ amount_____

Purpose
_____
_____
_____
_____
_____
_____
_____
_____
_____
_____
_____

Preparation
_____
_____
_____
_____
_____
_____
_____
_____
_____
_____
_____
_____
_____
_____

Notes ✏
_____
_____
_____
_____
_____
_____
_____
_____
_____
_____
_____
_____
_____

29

Love Factor

♡ ♡ ♡ ♡ ♡

How To Use

Blend Name

Purpose

_____
_____
_____
_____
_____
_____
_____
_____
_____
_____
_____

Ingredients ◇

Essential Oil (EO) and/or Hydrosol (H) Used

EO/H _____ # of drops _____
EO/H _____ # of drops _____
EO/H _____ # of drops _____
EO/H _____ # of drops _____
EO/H _____ # of drops _____
EO/H _____ # of drops _____

Carrier Oils (CO) Used

CO _____ amount_____
CO _____ amount_____
CO _____ amount_____

Notes ✏

_____
_____
_____
_____
_____
_____
_____
_____
_____
_____
_____
_____
_____
_____
30

Preparation

_____
_____
_____
_____
_____
_____
_____
_____
_____
_____
_____
_____
_____
_____
_____
_____
_____
_____

Blend Name

Love Factor

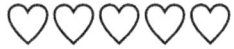

How To Use

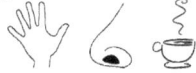

Ingredients 💧

Essential Oil (EO) and/or Hydrosol (H) Used

EO/H _____ # of drops _____
EO/H _____ # of drops _____
EO/H _____ # of drops _____
EO/H _____ # of drops _____
EO/H _____ # of drops _____
EO/H _____ # of drops _____

Carrier Oils (CO) Used

CO _____ amount_____
CO _____ amount_____
CO _____ amount_____

Preparation

_____
_____
_____
_____
_____
_____
_____
_____
_____
_____
_____
_____
_____
_____
_____
_____

Purpose

_____
_____
_____
_____
_____
_____
_____
_____
_____
_____
_____

Notes ✏️

_____
_____
_____
_____
_____
_____
_____
_____
_____
_____
_____
_____
_____

31

Love Factor

♡ ♡ ♡ ♡ ♡

How To Use

Blend Name

Purpose

_____
_____
_____
_____
_____
_____
_____
_____
_____
_____
_____

Ingredients ◌

Essential Oil (EO) and/or Hydrosol (H) Used

EO/H _____ # of drops _____
EO/H _____ # of drops _____
EO/H _____ # of drops _____
EO/H _____ # of drops _____
EO/H _____ # of drops _____
EO/H _____ # of drops _____

Carrier Oils (CO) Used

CO _____ amount_____
CO _____ amount_____
CO _____ amount_____

Notes ✏

Preparation

Blend Name

Love Factor
♡ ♡ ♡ ♡ ♡

How To Use
🖐 👃 ☕

Ingredients 💧

Essential Oil (EO) and/or Hydrosol (H) Used

EO/H _____ # of drops _____
EO/H _____ # of drops _____
EO/H _____ # of drops _____
EO/H _____ # of drops _____
EO/H _____ # of drops _____
EO/H _____ # of drops _____

Carrier Oils (CO) Used

CO _____ amount_____
CO _____ amount_____
CO _____ amount_____

Purpose

_____
_____
_____
_____
_____
_____
_____
_____
_____
_____
_____

Preparation

_____
_____
_____
_____
_____
_____
_____
_____
_____
_____
_____
_____
_____
_____
_____
_____
_____

Notes ✏

_____
_____
_____
_____
_____
_____
_____
_____
_____
_____
_____
_____
_____

Love Factor

♡ ♡ ♡ ♡ ♡

How To Use

Blend Name

Purpose

_____
_____
_____
_____
_____
_____
_____
_____
_____
_____
_____

Ingredients ⬡

Essential Oil (EO) and/or Hydrosol (H) Used

EO/H _____ # of drops _____
EO/H _____ # of drops _____
EO/H _____ # of drops _____
EO/H _____ # of drops _____
EO/H _____ # of drops _____
EO/H _____ # of drops _____

Carrier Oils (CO) Used

CO _____ amount_____
CO _____ amount_____
CO _____ amount_____

Notes ✏

_____
_____
_____
_____
_____
_____
_____
_____
_____
_____
_____
_____
_____
_____

Preparation

_____
_____
_____
_____
_____
_____
_____
_____
_____
_____
_____
_____
_____
_____
_____
_____
_____

Blend Name

Love Factor
♡♡♡♡♡

How To Use
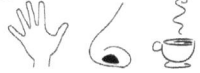

Ingredients 💧

Essential Oil (EO) and/or Hydrosol (H) Used

EO/H _____ # of drops _____

EO/H _____ # of drops _____

EO/H _____ # of drops _____

EO/H _____ # of drops _____

EO/H _____ # of drops _____

EO/H _____ # of drops _____

Carrier Oils (CO) Used

CO _____ amount_____

CO _____ amount_____

CO _____ amount_____

Purpose
_____
_____
_____
_____
_____
_____
_____
_____
_____
_____

Preparation
_____
_____
_____
_____
_____
_____
_____
_____
_____
_____
_____
_____
_____
_____
_____

Notes ✏
_____
_____
_____
_____
_____
_____
_____
_____
_____
_____
_____

Love Factor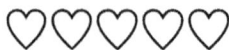
♡♡♡♡♡

How To Use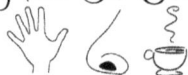

Blend Name

Purpose

_____
_____
_____
_____
_____
_____
_____
_____
_____
_____
_____

Ingredients ⬡

Essential Oil (EO) and/or Hydrosol (H) Used
EO/H _____ # of drops _____
EO/H _____ # of drops _____
EO/H _____ # of drops _____
EO/H _____ # of drops _____
EO/H _____ # of drops _____
EO/H _____ # of drops _____

Carrier Oils (CO) Used
CO _____ amount_____
CO _____ amount_____
CO _____ amount_____

Notes ✎

_____
_____
_____
_____
_____
_____
_____
_____
_____
_____
_____
_____
_____
_____

Preparation

_____
_____
_____
_____
_____
_____
_____
_____
_____
_____
_____
_____
_____
_____
_____
_____

Blend Name

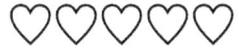
♡ ♡ ♡ ♡ ♡

How To Use
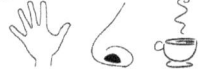

Ingredients ◌

Essential Oil (EO) and/or **Hydrosol (H) Used**

Purpose

_____

EO/H _____ # of drops _____ _____

EO/H _____ # of drops _____ _____

EO/H _____ # of drops _____ _____

EO/H _____ # of drops _____ _____

EO/H _____ # of drops _____ _____

EO/H _____ # of drops _____ _____

_____

Carrier Oils (CO) Used

_____

CO _____ amount_____ _____

CO _____ amount_____ _____

CO _____ amount_____ _____

Preparation

Notes ✏

_____ _____

_____ _____

_____ _____

_____ _____

_____ _____

_____ _____

_____ _____

_____ _____

_____ _____

_____ _____

_____ _____

_____ _____

_____ _____

_____ _____

_____ _____

_____ _____

Love Factor
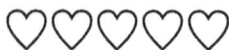
♡ ♡ ♡ ♡ ♡

How To Use
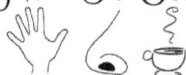

Blend Name

Purpose

_____
_____
_____
_____
_____
_____
_____
_____
_____
_____

Ingredients

Essential Oil (EO) and/or **Hydrosol (H) Used**

EO/H _____ # of drops _____
EO/H _____ # of drops _____
EO/H _____ # of drops _____
EO/H _____ # of drops _____
EO/H _____ # of drops _____
EO/H _____ # of drops _____

Carrier Oils (CO) Used

CO _____ amount_____
CO _____ amount_____
CO _____ amount_____

Notes

Preparation

Blend Name

Love Factor
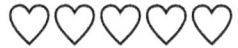

How To Use
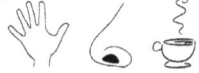

Ingredients ⬦

Purpose

Essential Oil (EO) and/or Hydrosol (H) Used _____

EO/H _____ # of drops _____ _____
EO/H _____ # of drops _____ _____
EO/H _____ # of drops _____ _____
EO/H _____ # of drops _____ _____
EO/H _____ # of drops _____ _____
EO/H _____ # of drops _____ _____

_____

Carrier Oils (CO) Used _____
CO _____ amount_____ _____
CO _____ amount_____ _____
CO _____ amount_____ _____

Preparation

Notes ✎

_____   _____
_____   _____
_____   _____
_____   _____
_____   _____
_____   _____
_____   _____
_____   _____
_____   _____
_____   _____
_____   _____
_____   _____
_____   _____
_____   _____
_____   _____
_____   _____
_____
                                    39
_____

Love Factor

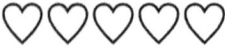

♡ ♡ ♡ ♡ ♡

How To Use

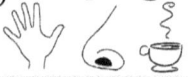

Blend Name

Purpose

_____
_____
_____
_____
_____
_____
_____
_____
_____
_____
_____

Ingredients ◊

Essential Oil (EO) and/or Hydrosol (H) Used

EO/H _____ # of drops _____
EO/H _____ # of drops _____
EO/H _____ # of drops _____
EO/H _____ # of drops _____
EO/H _____ # of drops _____
EO/H _____ # of drops _____

Carrier Oils (CO) Used

CO _____ amount_____
CO _____ amount_____
CO _____ amount_____

Notes ✏

_____
_____
_____
_____
_____
_____
_____
_____
_____
_____
_____
_____
_____

40

Preparation

_____
_____
_____
_____
_____
_____
_____
_____
_____
_____
_____
_____
_____
_____
_____
_____
_____

Blend Name

Love Factor
♡♡♡♡♡

How To Use
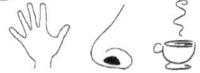

Ingredients

Essential Oil (EO) and/or Hydrosol (H) Used

EO/H _____ # of drops _____

EO/H _____ # of drops _____

EO/H _____ # of drops _____

EO/H _____ # of drops _____

EO/H _____ # of drops _____

EO/H _____ # of drops _____

Carrier Oils (CO) Used

CO _____ amount_____

CO _____ amount_____

CO _____ amount_____

Preparation

_____

_____

_____

_____

_____

_____

_____

_____

_____

_____

_____

_____

_____

_____

_____

Purpose

_____

_____

_____

_____

_____

_____

_____

_____

_____

_____

_____

Notes

_____

_____

_____

_____

_____

_____

_____

_____

_____

_____

_____

_____

_____

Love Factor

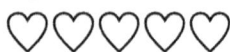
♡ ♡ ♡ ♡ ♡

How To Use

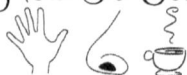

Blend Name

Purpose

_____
_____
_____
_____
_____
_____
_____
_____
_____
_____
_____
_____

Ingredients ⬯

Essential Oil (EO) and/or Hydrosol (H) Used
EO/H _____ # of drops _____
EO/H _____ # of drops _____
EO/H _____ # of drops _____
EO/H _____ # of drops _____
EO/H _____ # of drops _____
EO/H _____ # of drops _____

Carrier Oils (CO) Used
CO _____ amount_____
CO _____ amount_____
CO _____ amount_____

Notes ✏

_____
_____
_____
_____
_____
_____
_____
_____
_____
_____
_____
_____
_____
_____

Preparation

_____
_____
_____
_____
_____
_____
_____
_____
_____
_____
_____
_____
_____
_____
_____
_____
_____

Blend Name

Love Factor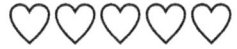
♡♡♡♡♡

How To Use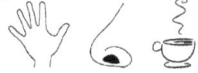

Ingredients ⬡

Purpose

Essential Oil (EO) and/or Hydrosol (H) Used _____

EO/H _____ # of drops _____ _____
EO/H _____ # of drops _____ _____
EO/H _____ # of drops _____ _____
EO/H _____ # of drops _____ _____
EO/H _____ # of drops _____ _____
EO/H _____ # of drops _____ _____

_____

Carrier Oils (CO) Used

_____
CO _____ amount_____ _____
CO _____ amount_____ _____
CO _____ amount_____ _____

Preparation

Notes ✏

_____ _____
_____ _____
_____ _____
_____ _____
_____ _____
_____ _____
_____ _____
_____ _____
_____ _____
_____ _____
_____ _____
_____ _____
_____ _____
_____ _____
_____ _____
_____ _____
_____ _____ 43
_____

Love Factor

♡ ♡ ♡ ♡ ♡

How To Use

Blend Name

Purpose

_____
_____
_____
_____
_____
_____
_____
_____
_____
_____
_____
_____

Ingredients 💧

Essential Oil (EO) and/or Hydrosol (H) Used
EO/H _____ # of drops _____
EO/H _____ # of drops _____
EO/H _____ # of drops _____
EO/H _____ # of drops _____
EO/H _____ # of drops _____
EO/H _____ # of drops _____

Carrier Oils (CO) Used
CO _____ amount_____
CO _____ amount_____
CO _____ amount_____

Notes ✏

_____
_____
_____
_____
_____
_____
_____
_____
_____
_____
_____
_____
_____
_____

Preparation

_____
_____
_____
_____
_____
_____
_____
_____
_____
_____
_____
_____
_____
_____
_____

Blend Name

Love Factor
♡ ♡ ♡ ♡ ♡

How To Use

Ingredients 💧

Essential Oil (EO) and/or Hydrosol (H) Used

EO/H _____ # of drops _____

EO/H _____ # of drops _____

EO/H _____ # of drops _____

EO/H _____ # of drops _____

EO/H _____ # of drops _____

EO/H _____ # of drops _____

Carrier Oils (CO) Used

CO _____ amount_____

CO _____ amount_____

CO _____ amount_____

Purpose

_____
_____
_____
_____
_____
_____
_____
_____
_____
_____
_____

Preparation

_____
_____
_____
_____
_____
_____
_____
_____
_____
_____
_____
_____
_____
_____
_____
_____

Notes ✏

_____
_____
_____
_____
_____
_____
_____
_____
_____
_____
_____
_____
_____

Love Factor

♡ ♡ ♡ ♡ ♡

How To Use

Blend Name

Purpose

_____
_____
_____
_____
_____
_____
_____
_____
_____
_____
_____

Ingredients ◯

Essential Oil (EO) and/or Hydrosol (H) Used

EO/H _____ # of drops _____
EO/H _____ # of drops _____
EO/H _____ # of drops _____
EO/H _____ # of drops _____
EO/H _____ # of drops _____
EO/H _____ # of drops _____

Carrier Oils (CO) Used

CO _____ amount_____
CO _____ amount_____
CO _____ amount_____

Notes ✐

_____
_____
_____
_____
_____
_____
_____
_____
_____
_____
_____
_____
_____
_____

Preparation

_____
_____
_____
_____
_____
_____
_____
_____
_____
_____
_____
_____
_____
_____
_____
_____

Blend Name

Love Factor
♡♡♡♡♡

How To Use
✋ 👃 ☕

Ingredients ◌

Essential Oil (EO) and/or Hydrosol (H) Used

EO/H _____ # of drops _____
EO/H _____ # of drops _____
EO/H _____ # of drops _____
EO/H _____ # of drops _____
EO/H _____ # of drops _____
EO/H _____ # of drops _____

Carrier Oils (CO) Used

CO _____ amount_____
CO _____ amount_____
CO _____ amount_____

Preparation
_____
_____
_____
_____
_____
_____
_____
_____
_____
_____
_____
_____
_____
_____
_____
_____
_____

Purpose
_____
_____
_____
_____
_____
_____
_____
_____
_____
_____
_____
_____

Notes ✏
_____
_____
_____
_____
_____
_____
_____
_____
_____
_____
_____
_____
_____
_____

47

Love Factor

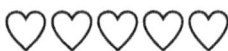
♡ ♡ ♡ ♡ ♡

How To Use

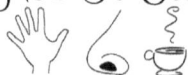

Blend Name

Purpose

_____
_____
_____
_____
_____
_____
_____
_____
_____
_____
_____
_____

Ingredients ⬡

Essential Oil (EO) and/or Hydrosol (H) Used
EO/H _____ # of drops _____
EO/H _____ # of drops _____
EO/H _____ # of drops _____
EO/H _____ # of drops _____
EO/H _____ # of drops _____
EO/H _____ # of drops _____

Carrier Oils (CO) Used
CO _____ amount_____
CO _____ amount_____
CO _____ amount_____

Notes ✏

_____
_____
_____
_____
_____
_____
_____
_____
_____
_____
_____
_____
_____

Preparation

_____
_____
_____
_____
_____
_____
_____
_____
_____
_____
_____
_____
_____
_____
_____

Blend Name

Love Factor
♡ ♡ ♡ ♡ ♡

How To Use
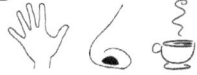

Ingredients 💧

Essential Oil (EO) and/or Hydrosol (H) Used

EO/H _____ # of drops _____
EO/H _____ # of drops _____
EO/H _____ # of drops _____
EO/H _____ # of drops _____
EO/H _____ # of drops _____
EO/H _____ # of drops _____

Carrier Oils (CO) Used

CO _____ amount_____
CO _____ amount_____
CO _____ amount_____

Purpose
_____
_____
_____
_____
_____
_____
_____
_____
_____
_____
_____

Preparation
_____
_____
_____
_____
_____
_____
_____
_____
_____
_____
_____
_____
_____
_____
_____
_____

Notes ✏
_____
_____
_____
_____
_____
_____
_____
_____
_____
_____
_____
_____
_____
_____
_____

Love Factor

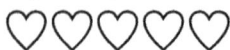

How To Use

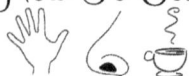

Blend Name

Purpose

_____
_____
_____
_____
_____
_____
_____
_____
_____
_____
_____

Ingredients ⬭

Essential Oil (EO) and/or Hydrosol (H) Used
EO/H _____ # of drops _____
EO/H _____ # of drops _____
EO/H _____ # of drops _____
EO/H _____ # of drops _____
EO/H _____ # of drops _____
EO/H _____ # of drops _____

Carrier Oils (CO) Used
CO _____ amount_____
CO _____ amount_____
CO _____ amount_____

Notes ✐

_____
_____
_____
_____
_____
_____
_____
_____
_____
_____
_____
_____
_____
_____

Preparation

_____
_____
_____
_____
_____
_____
_____
_____
_____
_____
_____
_____
_____
_____
_____

Blend Name

Love Factor
♡♡♡♡♡

How To Use

Ingredients ◯

Essential Oil (EO) and/or Hydrosol (H) Used

EO/H _____ # of drops _____
EO/H _____ # of drops _____
EO/H _____ # of drops _____
EO/H _____ # of drops _____
EO/H _____ # of drops _____
EO/H _____ # of drops _____

Carrier Oils (CO) Used

CO _____ amount_____
CO _____ amount_____
CO _____ amount_____

Purpose

_____
_____
_____
_____
_____
_____
_____
_____
_____
_____
_____

Preparation

_____
_____
_____
_____
_____
_____
_____
_____
_____
_____
_____
_____
_____
_____
_____
_____

Notes ✎

_____
_____
_____
_____
_____
_____
_____
_____
_____
_____
_____
_____
_____
_____

Love Factor

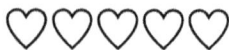

♡ ♡ ♡ ♡ ♡

How To Use

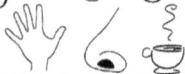

Blend Name

Purpose

_____
_____
_____
_____
_____
_____
_____
_____
_____
_____
_____
_____

Ingredients ⬡

Essential Oil (EO) and/or Hydrosol (H) Used

EO/H _____ # of drops _____
EO/H _____ # of drops _____
EO/H _____ # of drops _____
EO/H _____ # of drops _____
EO/H _____ # of drops _____
EO/H _____ # of drops _____

Carrier Oils (CO) Used

CO _____ amount_____
CO _____ amount_____
CO _____ amount_____

Notes ✏

_____
_____
_____
_____
_____
_____
_____
_____
_____
_____
_____
_____
_____
_____

Preparation

_____
_____
_____
_____
_____
_____
_____
_____
_____
_____
_____
_____
_____
_____
_____
_____
_____

Blend Name

Love Factor
♡♡♡♡♡

How To Use

Ingredients ◌

Essential Oil (EO) and/or Hydrosol (H) Used _____
EO/H _____ # of drops _____ _____
EO/H _____ # of drops _____ _____
EO/H _____ # of drops _____ _____
EO/H _____ # of drops _____ _____
EO/H _____ # of drops _____ _____
EO/H _____ # of drops _____ _____

Carrier Oils (CO) Used
CO _____ amount_____ _____
CO _____ amount_____ _____
CO _____ amount_____ _____

Purpose _____
_____
_____
_____
_____
_____
_____
_____
_____
_____
_____
_____

Preparation
_____
_____
_____
_____
_____
_____
_____
_____
_____
_____
_____
_____
_____
_____
_____
_____

Notes ✎
_____
_____
_____
_____
_____
_____
_____
_____
_____
_____
_____
_____
_____
_____
53

Love Factor

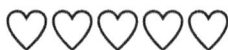

How To Use

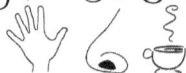

Blend Name

Purpose

_____
_____
_____
_____
_____
_____
_____
_____
_____
_____
_____

Ingredients ○

Essential Oil (EO) and/or Hydrosol (H) Used
EO/H _____ # of drops _____
EO/H _____ # of drops _____
EO/H _____ # of drops _____
EO/H _____ # of drops _____
EO/H _____ # of drops _____
EO/H _____ # of drops _____

Carrier Oils (CO) Used
CO _____ amount_____
CO _____ amount_____
CO _____ amount_____

Notes ✏

Preparation

Blend Name

Love Factor
♡♡♡♡♡

How To Use

Ingredients ○

Purpose

Essential Oil (EO) and/or Hydrosol (H) Used _____

EO/H _____ # of drops _____ _____
EO/H _____ # of drops _____ _____
EO/H _____ # of drops _____ _____
EO/H _____ # of drops _____ _____
EO/H _____ # of drops _____ _____
EO/H _____ # of drops _____ _____

_____

Carrier Oils (CO) Used

CO _____ amount_____ _____
CO _____ amount_____ _____
CO _____ amount_____ _____

Preparation

Notes ✏

_____   _____
_____   _____
_____   _____
_____   _____
_____   _____
_____   _____
_____   _____
_____   _____
_____   _____
_____   _____
_____   _____
_____   _____
_____   _____
_____   _____
_____   _____
_____   _____

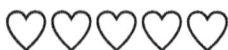Love Factor
♡ ♡ ♡ ♡ ♡

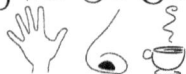How To Use

Blend Name

Purpose

_____
_____
_____
_____
_____
_____
_____
_____
_____
_____
_____

Ingredients 💧

Essential Oil (EO) and/or Hydrosol (H) Used
EO/H _____ # of drops _____
EO/H _____ # of drops _____
EO/H _____ # of drops _____
EO/H _____ # of drops _____
EO/H _____ # of drops _____
EO/H _____ # of drops _____

Carrier Oils (CO) Used
CO _____ amount_____
CO _____ amount_____
CO _____ amount_____

Notes ✏

_____
_____
_____
_____
_____
_____
_____
_____
_____
_____
_____
_____
_____
_____
56

Preparation

_____
_____
_____
_____
_____
_____
_____
_____
_____
_____
_____
_____
_____
_____
_____
_____
_____
_____

Blend Name

Love Factor

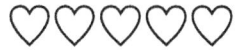

How To Use

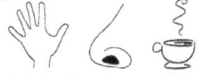

Ingredients

Purpose

Essential Oil (EO) and/or Hydrosol (H) Used _____

EO/H _____ # of drops _____ _____

EO/H _____ # of drops _____ _____

EO/H _____ # of drops _____ _____

EO/H _____ # of drops _____ _____

EO/H _____ # of drops _____ _____

EO/H _____ # of drops _____ _____

_____

Carrier Oils (CO) Used

CO _____ amount_____ _____

CO _____ amount_____ _____

CO _____ amount_____ _____

Preparation

Notes

_____ _____

_____ _____

_____ _____

_____ _____

_____ _____

_____ _____

_____ _____

_____ _____

_____ _____

_____ _____

_____ _____

_____ _____

_____ _____

_____ _____

_____ _____

_____ _____

Love Factor

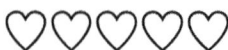

♡ ♡ ♡ ♡ ♡

How To Use

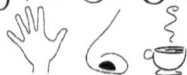

Blend Name

Purpose

_____
_____
_____
_____
_____
_____
_____
_____
_____
_____
_____

Ingredients ⬡

Essential Oil (EO) and/or Hydrosol (H) Used

EO/H _____ # of drops _____

EO/H _____ # of drops _____

EO/H _____ # of drops _____

EO/H _____ # of drops _____

EO/H _____ # of drops _____

EO/H _____ # of drops _____

Carrier Oils (CO) Used

CO _____ amount_____

CO _____ amount_____

CO _____ amount_____

Notes ✏

_____
_____
_____
_____
_____
_____
_____
_____
_____
_____
_____
_____
_____

58

Preparation

_____
_____
_____
_____
_____
_____
_____
_____
_____
_____
_____
_____
_____
_____
_____
_____
_____

Blend Name

Love Factor

♡ ♡ ♡ ♡ ♡

How To Use

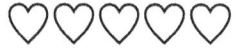

Ingredients

Essential Oil (EO) and/or Hydrosol (H) Used

EO/H _____ # of drops _____

EO/H _____ # of drops _____

EO/H _____ # of drops _____

EO/H _____ # of drops _____

EO/H _____ # of drops _____

EO/H _____ # of drops _____

Carrier Oils (CO) Used

CO _____ amount_____

CO _____ amount_____

CO _____ amount_____

Purpose

_____

_____

_____

_____

_____

_____

_____

_____

_____

_____

_____

Preparation

_____

_____

_____

_____

_____

_____

_____

_____

_____

_____

_____

_____

_____

_____

_____

_____

Notes

_____

_____

_____

_____

_____

_____

_____

_____

_____

_____

_____

_____

_____

59

Love Factor

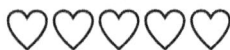

How To Use

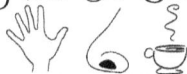

Blend Name

Purpose

_____
_____
_____
_____
_____
_____
_____
_____
_____
_____
_____

Ingredients

Essential Oil (EO) and/or Hydrosol (H) Used
EO/H _____ # of drops _____
EO/H _____ # of drops _____
EO/H _____ # of drops _____
EO/H _____ # of drops _____
EO/H _____ # of drops _____
EO/H _____ # of drops _____

Carrier Oils (CO) Used
CO _____ amount_____
CO _____ amount_____
CO _____ amount_____

Notes

_____
_____
_____
_____
_____
_____
_____
_____
_____
_____
_____
_____
_____
_____
_____

Preparation

_____
_____
_____
_____
_____
_____
_____
_____
_____
_____
_____
_____
_____
_____
_____
_____
_____

Blend Name

Love Factor
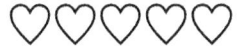

How To Use
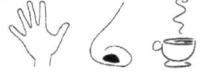

Ingredients

Essential Oil (EO) and/or Hydrosol (H) Used

EO/H _____ # of drops _____
EO/H _____ # of drops _____
EO/H _____ # of drops _____
EO/H _____ # of drops _____
EO/H _____ # of drops _____
EO/H _____ # of drops _____

Carrier Oils (CO) Used

CO _____ amount_____
CO _____ amount_____
CO _____ amount_____

Purpose

_____
_____
_____
_____
_____
_____
_____
_____
_____
_____
_____

Preparation

_____
_____
_____
_____
_____
_____
_____
_____
_____
_____
_____
_____
_____
_____
_____
_____

Notes

_____
_____
_____
_____
_____
_____
_____
_____
_____
_____
_____
_____

Love Factor

♡♡♡♡♡

How To Use

Blend Name

Purpose

_____
_____
_____
_____
_____
_____
_____
_____
_____
_____
_____
_____

Ingredients ⬦

Essential Oil (EO) and/or Hydrosol (H) Used
EO/H _____ # of drops _____
EO/H _____ # of drops _____
EO/H _____ # of drops _____
EO/H _____ # of drops _____
EO/H _____ # of drops _____
EO/H _____ # of drops _____

Carrier Oils (CO) Used
CO _____ amount_____
CO _____ amount_____
CO _____ amount_____

Notes ✏

_____
_____
_____
_____
_____
_____
_____
_____
_____
_____
_____
_____
_____
_____

Preparation

_____
_____
_____
_____
_____
_____
_____
_____
_____
_____
_____
_____
_____
_____
_____
_____
_____

Blend Name

Love Factor
♡ ♡ ♡ ♡ ♡

How To Use
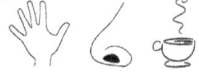

Ingredients ◌

Purpose

Essential Oil (EO) and/or Hydrosol (H) Used _____

EO/H _____ # of drops _____ _____
EO/H _____ # of drops _____ _____
EO/H _____ # of drops _____ _____
EO/H _____ # of drops _____ _____
EO/H _____ # of drops _____ _____
EO/H _____ # of drops _____ _____

_____

Carrier Oils (CO) Used

_____

CO _____ amount_____ _____
CO _____ amount_____ _____
CO _____ amount_____ _____

Preparation

Notes ✎

_____ _____
_____ _____
_____ _____
_____ _____
_____ _____
_____ _____
_____ _____
_____ _____
_____ _____
_____ _____
_____ _____
_____ _____
_____ _____
_____ _____

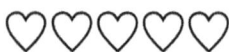

Love Factor
♡ ♡ ♡ ♡ ♡

How To Use
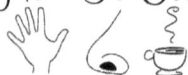

Blend Name

Purpose

_____
_____
_____
_____
_____
_____
_____
_____
_____
_____

Ingredients ◯

Essential Oil (EO) and/or Hydrosol (H) Used
EO/H _____ # of drops _____
EO/H _____ # of drops _____
EO/H _____ # of drops _____
EO/H _____ # of drops _____
EO/H _____ # of drops _____
EO/H _____ # of drops _____

Carrier Oils (CO) Used
CO _____ amount_____
CO _____ amount_____
CO _____ amount_____

Notes ✏

_____
_____
_____
_____
_____
_____
_____
_____
_____
_____
_____
_____
_____

Preparation

_____
_____
_____
_____
_____
_____
_____
_____
_____
_____
_____
_____
_____
_____
_____

Blend Name

Love Factor
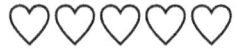

How To Use
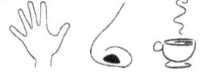

Ingredients ○

Purpose

Essential Oil (EO) and/or Hydrosol (H) Used _____

EO/H _____ # of drops _____ _____
EO/H _____ # of drops _____ _____
EO/H _____ # of drops _____ _____
EO/H _____ # of drops _____ _____
EO/H _____ # of drops _____ _____
EO/H _____ # of drops _____ _____

_____

Carrier Oils (CO) Used

_____

CO _____ amount_____ _____
CO _____ amount_____ _____
CO _____ amount_____ _____

Preparation

Notes ✏

_____ _____
_____ _____
_____ _____
_____ _____
_____ _____
_____ _____
_____ _____
_____ _____
_____ _____
_____ _____
_____ _____
_____ _____
_____ _____
_____ _____
_____ _____

Love Factor

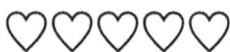

♡ ♡ ♡ ♡ ♡

How To Use

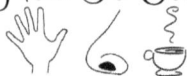

Blend Name

Purpose

_____
_____
_____
_____
_____
_____
_____
_____
_____
_____
_____

Ingredients ○

Essential Oil (EO) and/or Hydrosol (H) Used
EO/H _____ # of drops _____
EO/H _____ # of drops _____
EO/H _____ # of drops _____
EO/H _____ # of drops _____
EO/H _____ # of drops _____
EO/H _____ # of drops _____

Carrier Oils (CO) Used
CO _____ amount_____
CO _____ amount_____
CO _____ amount_____

Notes ✏

_____
_____
_____
_____
_____
_____
_____
_____
_____
_____
_____
_____
_____

Preparation

_____
_____
_____
_____
_____
_____
_____
_____
_____
_____
_____
_____
_____
_____
_____
_____
_____

Blend Name

Love Factor
♡♡♡♡♡

How To Use

Ingredients ◊

Essential Oil (EO) and/or Hydrosol (H) Used _____

EO/H _____	# of drops _____	_____
EO/H _____	# of drops _____	_____
EO/H _____	# of drops _____	_____
EO/H _____	# of drops _____	_____
EO/H _____	# of drops _____	_____
EO/H _____	# of drops _____	_____

Carrier Oils (CO) Used

CO _____	amount_____	_____
CO _____	amount_____	_____
CO _____	amount_____	_____

Purpose

_____

Preparation

_____
_____
_____
_____
_____
_____
_____
_____
_____
_____
_____
_____
_____
_____
_____
_____

Notes ✎

_____
_____
_____
_____
_____
_____
_____
_____
_____
_____
_____
_____
_____
_____

Love Factor

♡ ♡ ♡ ♡ ♡

How To Use

Blend Name

Purpose

_____
_____
_____
_____
_____
_____
_____
_____

_____
_____
_____

Ingredients ◊

Essential Oil (EO) and/or Hydrosol (H) Used
EO/H _____ # of drops _____
EO/H _____ # of drops _____
EO/H _____ # of drops _____
EO/H _____ # of drops _____
EO/H _____ # of drops _____
EO/H _____ # of drops _____

Carrier Oils (CO) Used
CO _____ amount_____
CO _____ amount_____
CO _____ amount_____

Notes ✏

_____
_____
_____
_____
_____
_____
_____
_____
_____
_____
_____
_____
_____
_____
68

Preparation

_____
_____
_____
_____
_____
_____
_____
_____
_____
_____
_____
_____
_____
_____
_____
_____
_____
_____

Blend Name

Love Factor
♡ ♡ ♡ ♡ ♡

How To Use
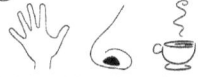

Ingredients 💧

Essential Oil (EO) and/or Hydrosol (H) Used

EO/H _____ # of drops _____

EO/H _____ # of drops _____

EO/H _____ # of drops _____

EO/H _____ # of drops _____

EO/H _____ # of drops _____

EO/H _____ # of drops _____

Carrier Oils (CO) Used

CO _____ amount_____

CO _____ amount_____

CO _____ amount_____

Purpose
_____
_____
_____
_____
_____
_____
_____
_____
_____
_____
_____
_____

Preparation

_____
_____
_____
_____
_____
_____
_____
_____
_____
_____
_____
_____
_____
_____
_____
_____

Notes ✏️
_____
_____
_____
_____
_____
_____
_____
_____
_____
_____
_____
_____

Love Factor
♡ ♡ ♡ ♡ ♡

Blend Name

How To Use

Purpose

_____
_____
_____
_____
_____
_____
_____
_____
_____
_____
_____

Ingredients ⬤

Essential Oil (EO) and/or Hydrosol (H) Used
EO/H _____ # of drops _____
EO/H _____ # of drops _____
EO/H _____ # of drops _____
EO/H _____ # of drops _____
EO/H _____ # of drops _____
EO/H _____ # of drops _____

Carrier Oils (CO) Used
CO _____ amount_____
CO _____ amount_____
CO _____ amount_____

Notes ✏

_____
_____
_____
_____
_____
_____
_____
_____
_____
_____
_____
_____
_____
_____
_____

Preparation

_____
_____
_____
_____
_____
_____
_____
_____
_____
_____
_____
_____
_____
_____
_____
_____

Blend Name

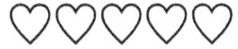

How To Use

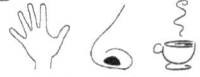

Ingredients ⬡

Purpose

Essential Oil (EO) and/or Hydrosol (H) Used _____
EO/H _____ # of drops _____ _____
EO/H _____ # of drops _____ _____
EO/H _____ # of drops _____ _____
EO/H _____ # of drops _____ _____
EO/H _____ # of drops _____ _____
EO/H _____ # of drops _____ _____

_____

Carrier Oils (CO) Used   _____
CO _____ amount_____ _____
CO _____ amount_____ _____
CO _____ amount_____ _____

Preparation   Notes ✎

_____ _____
_____ _____
_____ _____
_____ _____
_____ _____
_____ _____
_____ _____
_____ _____
_____ _____
_____ _____
_____ _____
_____ _____
_____ _____
_____ _____
_____ _____
_____ _____
_____ _____

Love Factor

♡ ♡ ♡ ♡ ♡

How To Use

Blend Name

Purpose

_____
_____
_____
_____
_____
_____
_____
_____
_____
_____

Ingredients ◊

Essential Oil (EO) and/or Hydrosol (H) Used

EO/H _____ # of drops _____
EO/H _____ # of drops _____
EO/H _____ # of drops _____
EO/H _____ # of drops _____
EO/H _____ # of drops _____
EO/H _____ # of drops _____

Carrier Oils (CO) Used

CO _____ amount_____
CO _____ amount_____
CO _____ amount_____

Notes ✏

_____
_____
_____
_____
_____
_____
_____
_____
_____
_____
_____
_____
_____
_____

72

Preparation

_____
_____
_____
_____
_____
_____
_____
_____
_____
_____
_____
_____
_____
_____
_____
_____

Blend Name

Love Factor
♡♡♡♡♡

How To Use
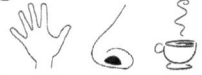

Ingredients ⬡

Essential Oil (EO) and/or Hydrosol (H) Used

EO/H _____ # of drops _____
EO/H _____ # of drops _____
EO/H _____ # of drops _____
EO/H _____ # of drops _____
EO/H _____ # of drops _____
EO/H _____ # of drops _____

Carrier Oils (CO) Used

CO _____ amount_____
CO _____ amount_____
CO _____ amount_____

Purpose
_____
_____
_____
_____
_____
_____
_____
_____
_____
_____
_____
_____

Preparation
_____
_____
_____
_____
_____
_____
_____
_____
_____
_____
_____
_____
_____
_____
_____
_____

Notes ✏
_____
_____
_____
_____
_____
_____
_____
_____
_____
_____
_____
_____
_____
_____
_____

Love Factor

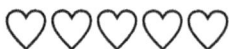
♡ ♡ ♡ ♡ ♡

How To Use

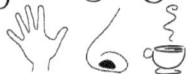

Blend Name

Purpose

_____
_____
_____
_____
_____
_____
_____
_____
_____
_____
_____
_____

Ingredients ◇

Essential Oil (EO) and/or Hydrosol (H) Used

EO/H _____ # of drops _____
EO/H _____ # of drops _____
EO/H _____ # of drops _____
EO/H _____ # of drops _____
EO/H _____ # of drops _____
EO/H _____ # of drops _____

Carrier Oils (CO) Used

CO _____ amount_____
CO _____ amount_____
CO _____ amount_____

Notes ✏

_____
_____
_____
_____
_____
_____
_____
_____
_____
_____
_____
_____
_____
_____

Preparation

_____
_____
_____
_____
_____
_____
_____
_____
_____
_____
_____
_____
_____
_____
_____
_____
_____
_____

Blend Name

Love Factor
♡ ♡ ♡ ♡ ♡

How To Use
🖐 👃 ☕

Ingredients 💧

Essential Oil (EO) and/or Hydrosol (H) Used

EO/H _____ # of drops _____
EO/H _____ # of drops _____
EO/H _____ # of drops _____
EO/H _____ # of drops _____
EO/H _____ # of drops _____
EO/H _____ # of drops _____

Carrier Oils (CO) Used

CO _____ amount_____
CO _____ amount_____
CO _____ amount_____

Purpose

_____
_____
_____
_____
_____
_____
_____
_____
_____
_____
_____

Preparation

_____
_____
_____
_____
_____
_____
_____
_____
_____
_____
_____
_____
_____
_____
_____
_____
_____

Notes ✏

_____
_____
_____
_____
_____
_____
_____
_____
_____
_____
_____
_____
_____
_____

Love Factor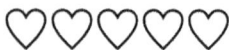
♡ ♡ ♡ ♡ ♡

How To Use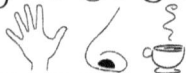

Blend Name

Purpose

_____
_____
_____
_____
_____
_____
_____

_____
_____
_____
_____

Ingredients ⬦

Essential Oil (EO) and/or Hydrosol (H) Used
EO/H _____ # of drops _____
EO/H _____ # of drops _____
EO/H _____ # of drops _____
EO/H _____ # of drops _____
EO/H _____ # of drops _____
EO/H _____ # of drops _____

Carrier Oils (CO) Used
CO _____ amount_____
CO _____ amount_____
CO _____ amount_____

Notes ✏

_____
_____
_____
_____
_____
_____
_____
_____
_____
_____
_____
_____
_____
_____
76

Preparation

_____
_____
_____
_____
_____
_____
_____
_____
_____
_____
_____
_____
_____
_____
_____
_____
_____

Blend Name

Love Factor

♡♡♡♡♡

How To Use

Ingredients ◯

Purpose

Essential Oil (EO) and/or Hydrosol (H) Used _____

EO/H _____ # of drops _____ _____

EO/H _____ # of drops _____ _____

EO/H _____ # of drops _____ _____

EO/H _____ # of drops _____ _____

EO/H _____ # of drops _____ _____

EO/H _____ # of drops _____ _____

_____

Carrier Oils (CO) Used

_____

CO _____ amount_____ _____

CO _____ amount_____ _____

CO _____ amount_____ _____

Preparation

Notes ✏

_____ _____

_____ _____

_____ _____

_____ _____

_____ _____

_____ _____

_____ _____

_____ _____

_____ _____

_____ _____

_____ _____

_____ _____

_____ _____

_____ _____

_____ _____

_____ 77

_____

Love Factor
♡♡♡♡♡

How To Use

Blend Name

Purpose

_____
_____
_____
_____
_____
_____
_____
_____
_____
_____
_____
_____

Ingredients 💧

Essential Oil (EO) and/or Hydrosol (H) Used
EO/H _____ # of drops _____
EO/H _____ # of drops _____
EO/H _____ # of drops _____
EO/H _____ # of drops _____
EO/H _____ # of drops _____
EO/H _____ # of drops _____

Carrier Oils (CO) Used
CO _____ amount_____
CO _____ amount_____
CO _____ amount_____

Notes ✏️

_____
_____
_____
_____
_____
_____
_____
_____
_____
_____
_____
_____
_____
_____

Preparation

_____
_____
_____
_____
_____
_____
_____
_____
_____
_____
_____
_____
_____
_____
_____
_____

Blend Name

Love Factor
♡♡♡♡♡

How To Use

Ingredients ◌

Essential Oil (EO) and/or Hydrosol (H) Used

EO/H _____ # of drops _____
EO/H _____ # of drops _____
EO/H _____ # of drops _____
EO/H _____ # of drops _____
EO/H _____ # of drops _____
EO/H _____ # of drops _____

Carrier Oils (CO) Used

CO _____ amount_____
CO _____ amount_____
CO _____ amount_____

Preparation

_____
_____
_____
_____
_____
_____
_____
_____
_____
_____
_____
_____
_____
_____
_____

Purpose

_____
_____
_____
_____
_____
_____
_____
_____
_____
_____

Notes ✏

_____
_____
_____
_____
_____
_____
_____
_____
_____
_____
_____
_____
_____
_____
_____

Love Factor

♡ ♡ ♡ ♡ ♡

How To Use

Purpose

_____
_____
_____
_____
_____
_____
_____
_____
_____
_____
_____
_____

Blend Name

Ingredients ⬡

Essential Oil (EO) and/or Hydrosol (H) Used

EO/H _____ # of drops _____
EO/H _____ # of drops _____
EO/H _____ # of drops _____
EO/H _____ # of drops _____
EO/H _____ # of drops _____
EO/H _____ # of drops _____

Carrier Oils (CO) Used

CO _____ amount_____
CO _____ amount_____
CO _____ amount_____

Notes ✏

_____
_____
_____
_____
_____
_____
_____
_____
_____
_____
_____
_____
_____
_____

Preparation

_____
_____
_____
_____
_____
_____
_____
_____
_____
_____
_____
_____
_____
_____
_____
_____
_____

Blend Name

Love Factor

♡♡♡♡♡

How To Use

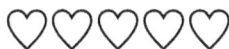

Ingredients

Essential Oil (EO) and/or Hydrosol (H) Used

EO/H _____ # of drops _____
EO/H _____ # of drops _____
EO/H _____ # of drops _____
EO/H _____ # of drops _____
EO/H _____ # of drops _____
EO/H _____ # of drops _____

Carrier Oils (CO) Used

CO _____ amount_____
CO _____ amount_____
CO _____ amount_____

Preparation

_____
_____
_____
_____
_____
_____
_____
_____
_____
_____
_____
_____
_____
_____
_____
_____

Purpose

_____
_____
_____
_____
_____
_____
_____
_____
_____
_____
_____

Notes

_____
_____
_____
_____
_____
_____
_____
_____
_____
_____
_____
_____
_____

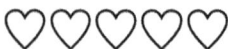

Love Factor

♡ ♡ ♡ ♡ ♡

How To Use

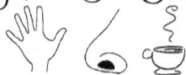

Blend Name

Purpose

_____
_____
_____
_____
_____
_____
_____
_____
_____
_____

Ingredients ◊

Essential Oil (EO) and/or Hydrosol (H) Used

EO/H _____ # of drops _____
EO/H _____ # of drops _____
EO/H _____ # of drops _____
EO/H _____ # of drops _____
EO/H _____ # of drops _____
EO/H _____ # of drops _____

Carrier Oils (CO) Used

CO _____ amount_____
CO _____ amount_____
CO _____ amount_____

Notes 🖊

_____
_____
_____
_____
_____
_____
_____
_____
_____
_____
_____
_____
_____
_____

82

Preparation

_____
_____
_____
_____
_____
_____
_____
_____
_____
_____
_____
_____
_____
_____
_____
_____

Blend Name

Love Factor
♡♡♡♡♡

How To Use
🖐 👃 ☕

Ingredients ○

Essential Oil (EO) and/or Hydrosol (H) Used _____

EO/H _____ # of drops _____

EO/H _____ # of drops _____

EO/H _____ # of drops _____

EO/H _____ # of drops _____

EO/H _____ # of drops _____

EO/H _____ # of drops _____

Carrier Oils (CO) Used

CO _____ amount_____

CO _____ amount_____

CO _____ amount_____

Purpose
_____
_____
_____
_____
_____
_____
_____
_____
_____
_____
_____
_____

Preparation
_____
_____
_____
_____
_____
_____
_____
_____
_____
_____
_____
_____
_____
_____
_____
_____

Notes ✏
_____
_____
_____
_____
_____
_____
_____
_____
_____
_____
_____
_____
_____

Love Factor

♡ ♡ ♡ ♡ ♡

How To Use

Blend Name

Purpose

_____
_____
_____
_____
_____
_____
_____
_____
_____
_____
_____

Ingredients

Essential Oil (EO) and/or Hydrosol (H) Used

EO/H _____ # of drops _____
EO/H _____ # of drops _____
EO/H _____ # of drops _____
EO/H _____ # of drops _____
EO/H _____ # of drops _____
EO/H _____ # of drops _____

Carrier Oils (CO) Used

CO _____ amount_____
CO _____ amount_____
CO _____ amount_____

Notes

_____
_____
_____
_____
_____
_____
_____
_____
_____
_____
_____
_____
_____
_____

Preparation

_____
_____
_____
_____
_____
_____
_____
_____
_____
_____
_____
_____
_____
_____
_____

Blend Name

Love Factor
♡ ♡ ♡ ♡ ♡

How To Use

Ingredients ⬦

Purpose

Essential Oil (EO) and/or Hydrosol (H) Used _____

EO/H _____ # of drops _____ _____

EO/H _____ # of drops _____ _____

EO/H _____ # of drops _____ _____

EO/H _____ # of drops _____ _____

EO/H _____ # of drops _____ _____

EO/H _____ # of drops _____ _____

_____

Carrier Oils (CO) Used

CO _____ amount_____ _____

CO _____ amount_____ _____

CO _____ amount_____ _____

Preparation

Notes ✏

_____ _____

_____ _____

_____ _____

_____ _____

_____ _____

_____ _____

_____ _____

_____ _____

_____ _____

_____ _____

_____ _____

_____ _____

_____ _____

_____ _____

_____ _____

_____ _____

Love Factor
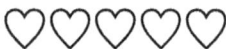

How To Use
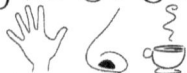

Blend Name

Purpose

_____
_____
_____
_____
_____
_____
_____
_____
_____
_____
_____

Ingredients ◊

Essential Oil (EO) and/or **Hydrosol (H) Used**

EO/H _____ # of drops _____
EO/H _____ # of drops _____
EO/H _____ # of drops _____
EO/H _____ # of drops _____
EO/H _____ # of drops _____
EO/H _____ # of drops _____

Carrier Oils (CO) Used

CO _____ amount_____
CO _____ amount_____
CO _____ amount_____

Notes ✏

_____
_____
_____
_____
_____
_____
_____
_____
_____
_____
_____
_____
_____

Preparation

_____
_____
_____
_____
_____
_____
_____
_____
_____
_____
_____
_____
_____
_____
_____
_____
_____

Blend Name

Love Factor
♡♡♡♡♡

How To Use
🖐 👃 ☕

Ingredients 💧

Purpose

Essential Oil (EO) and/or Hydrosol (H) Used _____

EO/H _____ # of drops _____ _____
EO/H _____ # of drops _____ _____
EO/H _____ # of drops _____ _____
EO/H _____ # of drops _____ _____
EO/H _____ # of drops _____ _____
EO/H _____ # of drops _____ _____

_____

Carrier Oils (CO) Used

_____
CO _____ amount _____ _____
CO _____ amount _____ _____
CO _____ amount _____ _____

Preparation

Notes ✏️

_____ _____
_____ _____
_____ _____
_____ _____
_____ _____
_____ _____
_____ _____
_____ _____
_____ _____
_____ _____
_____ _____
_____ _____
_____ _____
_____ _____
_____ _____

Love Factor

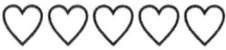

♡ ♡ ♡ ♡ ♡

How To Use

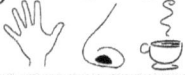

Blend Name

Purpose

_____
_____
_____
_____
_____
_____
_____
_____
_____
_____
_____
_____

Ingredients ◊

Essential Oil (EO) and/or Hydrosol (H) Used
EO/H _____ # of drops _____
EO/H _____ # of drops _____
EO/H _____ # of drops _____
EO/H _____ # of drops _____
EO/H _____ # of drops _____
EO/H _____ # of drops _____

Carrier Oils (CO) Used
CO _____ amount_____
CO _____ amount_____
CO _____ amount_____

Notes ✏

_____
_____
_____
_____
_____
_____
_____
_____
_____
_____
_____
_____
_____
_____

Preparation

_____
_____
_____
_____
_____
_____
_____
_____
_____
_____
_____
_____
_____
_____
_____
_____
_____
_____

Blend Name

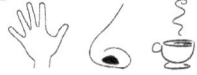
Ingredients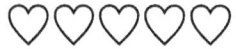

Purpose

Essential Oil (EO) and/or Hydrosol (H) Used _____

EO/H _____ # of drops _____ _____
EO/H _____ # of drops _____ _____
EO/H _____ # of drops _____ _____
EO/H _____ # of drops _____ _____
EO/H _____ # of drops _____ _____
EO/H _____ # of drops _____ _____

_____

Carrier Oils (CO) Used   _____
CO _____ amount_____ _____
CO _____ amount_____ _____
CO _____ amount_____ _____

Preparation

Notes ✏

_____   _____
_____   _____
_____   _____
_____   _____
_____   _____
_____   _____
_____   _____
_____   _____
_____   _____
_____   _____
_____   _____
_____   _____
_____   _____

Love Factor

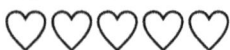

How To Use

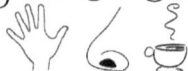

Blend Name

Purpose

_____
_____
_____
_____
_____
_____
_____
_____
_____
_____
_____
_____

Ingredients ◊

Essential Oil (EO) and/or **Hydrosol (H) Used**
EO/H _____ # of drops _____
EO/H _____ # of drops _____
EO/H _____ # of drops _____
EO/H _____ # of drops _____
EO/H _____ # of drops _____
EO/H _____ # of drops _____

Carrier Oils (CO) Used
CO _____ amount_____
CO _____ amount_____
CO _____ amount_____

Notes ✏

_____
_____
_____
_____
_____
_____
_____
_____
_____
_____
_____
_____
_____
_____

90

Preparation

_____
_____
_____
_____
_____
_____
_____
_____
_____
_____
_____
_____
_____
_____
_____
_____
_____

Blend Name

Love Factor
♡ ♡ ♡ ♡ ♡

How To Use
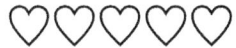
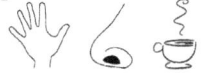

Ingredients ◯

Essential Oil (EO) and/or Hydrosol (H) Used

EO/H _____ # of drops _____
EO/H _____ # of drops _____
EO/H _____ # of drops _____
EO/H _____ # of drops _____
EO/H _____ # of drops _____
EO/H _____ # of drops _____

Carrier Oils (CO) Used

CO _____ amount_____
CO _____ amount_____
CO _____ amount_____

Purpose

_____
_____
_____
_____
_____
_____
_____
_____
_____
_____
_____
_____

Preparation

_____
_____
_____
_____
_____
_____
_____
_____
_____
_____
_____
_____
_____
_____
_____
_____
_____

Notes ✏

_____
_____
_____
_____
_____
_____
_____
_____
_____
_____
_____
_____
_____
_____

Love Factor

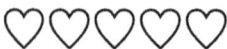

How To Use

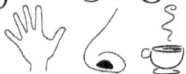

Blend Name

Purpose

_____
_____
_____
_____
_____
_____
_____
_____
_____
_____
_____

Ingredients ◇

Essential Oil (EO) and/or Hydrosol (H) Used

EO/H _____ # of drops _____
EO/H _____ # of drops _____
EO/H _____ # of drops _____
EO/H _____ # of drops _____
EO/H _____ # of drops _____
EO/H _____ # of drops _____

Carrier Oils (CO) Used

CO _____ amount_____
CO _____ amount_____
CO _____ amount_____

Notes ✏

_____
_____
_____
_____
_____
_____
_____
_____
_____
_____
_____
_____
_____
_____

Preparation

_____
_____
_____
_____
_____
_____
_____
_____
_____
_____
_____
_____
_____
_____
_____
_____
_____
_____

Blend Name

Love Factor
♡ ♡ ♡ ♡ ♡

How To Use

Ingredients ◌

Essential Oil (EO) and/or **Hydrosol (H) Used**

EO/H _____	# of drops _____	_____
EO/H _____	# of drops _____	_____
EO/H _____	# of drops _____	_____
EO/H _____	# of drops _____	_____
EO/H _____	# of drops _____	_____
EO/H _____	# of drops _____	_____

Purpose

_____

Carrier Oils (CO) Used

CO _____	amount_____	_____
CO _____	amount_____	_____
CO _____	amount_____	_____

Preparation

_____
_____
_____
_____
_____
_____
_____
_____
_____
_____
_____
_____
_____
_____
_____
_____

Notes ✎

_____
_____
_____
_____
_____
_____
_____
_____
_____
_____
_____
_____
_____
_____

Love Factor

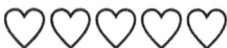

How To Use

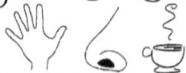

Blend Name

Purpose

_____
_____
_____
_____
_____
_____
_____
_____
_____
_____
_____

Ingredients

Essential Oil (EO) and/or Hydrosol (H) Used
EO/H _____ # of drops _____
EO/H _____ # of drops _____
EO/H _____ # of drops _____
EO/H _____ # of drops _____
EO/H _____ # of drops _____
EO/H _____ # of drops _____

Carrier Oils (CO) Used
CO _____ amount_____
CO _____ amount_____
CO _____ amount_____

Notes

_____
_____
_____
_____
_____
_____
_____
_____
_____
_____
_____
_____
_____
_____

Preparation

_____
_____
_____
_____
_____
_____
_____
_____
_____
_____
_____
_____
_____
_____
_____
_____
_____
_____

Blend Name

Love Factor
♡♡♡♡♡

How To Use

Ingredients ◌

Essential Oil (EO) and/or Hydrosol (H) Used

EO/H _____ # of drops _____
EO/H _____ # of drops _____
EO/H _____ # of drops _____
EO/H _____ # of drops _____
EO/H _____ # of drops _____
EO/H _____ # of drops _____

Carrier Oils (CO) Used

CO _____ amount_____
CO _____ amount_____
CO _____ amount_____

Purpose

_____
_____
_____
_____
_____
_____
_____
_____
_____
_____
_____

Preparation

_____
_____
_____
_____
_____
_____
_____
_____
_____
_____
_____
_____
_____
_____
_____
_____

Notes ✏

_____
_____
_____
_____
_____
_____
_____
_____
_____
_____
_____
_____
_____
_____

Love Factor

♡ ♡ ♡ ♡ ♡

How To Use

Purpose

_____
_____
_____
_____
_____
_____
_____
_____
_____
_____
_____

Blend Name

Ingredients ◊

Essential Oil (EO) and/or Hydrosol (H) Used
EO/H _____ # of drops _____
EO/H _____ # of drops _____
EO/H _____ # of drops _____
EO/H _____ # of drops _____
EO/H _____ # of drops _____
EO/H _____ # of drops _____

Carrier Oils (CO) Used
CO _____ amount_____
CO _____ amount_____
CO _____ amount_____

Notes ✏

_____
_____
_____
_____
_____
_____
_____
_____
_____
_____
_____
_____
_____
_____

Preparation

_____
_____
_____
_____
_____
_____
_____
_____
_____
_____
_____
_____
_____
_____
_____
_____
_____

Blend Name

Love Factor

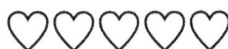

How To Use

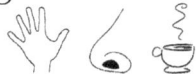

Ingredients 💧

Essential Oil (EO) and/or Hydrosol (H) Used _____

EO/H _____ # of drops _____ _____

EO/H _____ # of drops _____ _____

EO/H _____ # of drops _____ _____

EO/H _____ # of drops _____ _____

EO/H _____ # of drops _____ _____

EO/H _____ # of drops _____ _____

Purpose

_____

Carrier Oils (CO) Used

CO _____ amount_____ _____

CO _____ amount_____ _____

CO _____ amount_____ _____

Preparation

_____

_____

_____

_____

_____

_____

_____

_____

_____

_____

_____

_____

_____

_____

_____

Notes ✏️

_____

_____

_____

_____

_____

_____

_____

_____

_____

_____

_____

_____

_____

_____

Love Factor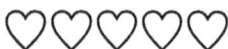
♡ ♡ ♡ ♡ ♡

How To Use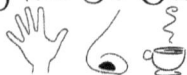

Blend Name

Purpose

_____
_____
_____
_____
_____
_____
_____

_____
_____
_____
_____

Ingredients ⬡

Essential Oil (EO) and/or Hydrosol (H) Used

EO/H _____ # of drops _____
EO/H _____ # of drops _____
EO/H _____ # of drops _____
EO/H _____ # of drops _____
EO/H _____ # of drops _____
EO/H _____ # of drops _____

Carrier Oils (CO) Used

CO _____ amount_____
CO _____ amount_____
CO _____ amount_____

Notes ✏

_____
_____
_____
_____
_____
_____
_____
_____
_____
_____
_____
_____
_____
_____

Preparation

_____
_____
_____
_____
_____
_____
_____
_____
_____
_____
_____
_____
_____
_____
_____
_____
_____
_____
_____

Blend Name

Love Factor
♡ ♡ ♡ ♡ ♡

How To Use

Ingredients

Essential Oil (EO) and/or Hydrosol (H) Used _____

EO/H _____ # of drops _____ _____
EO/H _____ # of drops _____ _____
EO/H _____ # of drops _____ _____
EO/H _____ # of drops _____ _____
EO/H _____ # of drops _____ _____
EO/H _____ # of drops _____ _____

Purpose
_____
_____
_____
_____
_____
_____
_____

Carrier Oils (CO) Used

CO _____ amount _____ _____
CO _____ amount _____ _____
CO _____ amount _____ _____

Preparation
_____
_____
_____
_____
_____
_____
_____
_____
_____
_____
_____
_____
_____
_____
_____
_____

Notes
_____
_____
_____
_____
_____
_____
_____
_____
_____
_____
_____
_____
_____
_____

Love Factor

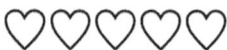

How To Use

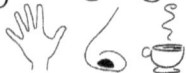

Blend Name

Purpose

_____
_____
_____
_____
_____
_____
_____
_____
_____
_____

Ingredients ⬡

Essential Oil (EO) and/or Hydrosol (H) Used

EO/H _____ # of drops _____
EO/H _____ # of drops _____
EO/H _____ # of drops _____
EO/H _____ # of drops _____
EO/H _____ # of drops _____
EO/H _____ # of drops _____

Carrier Oils (CO) Used

CO _____ amount_____
CO _____ amount_____
CO _____ amount_____

Notes ✏

_____
_____
_____
_____
_____
_____
_____
_____
_____
_____
_____
_____
_____
_____

100

Preparation

_____
_____
_____
_____
_____
_____
_____
_____
_____
_____
_____
_____
_____
_____
_____
_____

Blend Name

Love Factor

♡♡♡♡♡

How To Use

Ingredients ◯

Purpose

Essential Oil (EO) and/or Hydrosol (H) Used _____

EO/H _____ # of drops _____ _____
EO/H _____ # of drops _____ _____
EO/H _____ # of drops _____ _____
EO/H _____ # of drops _____ _____
EO/H _____ # of drops _____ _____
EO/H _____ # of drops _____ _____

Carrier Oils (CO) Used

CO _____ amount_____ _____
CO _____ amount_____ _____
CO _____ amount_____ _____

Preparation

Notes ✐

_____ _____
_____ _____
_____ _____
_____ _____
_____ _____
_____ _____
_____ _____
_____ _____
_____ _____
_____ _____
_____ _____
_____ _____
_____ _____
_____ _____

Love Factor

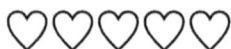

How To Use

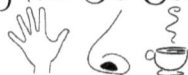

Blend Name

Purpose

_____
_____
_____
_____
_____
_____
_____

_____
_____
_____
_____

Ingredients

Essential Oil (EO) and/or Hydrosol (H) Used

EO/H _____ # of drops _____
EO/H _____ # of drops _____
EO/H _____ # of drops _____
EO/H _____ # of drops _____
EO/H _____ # of drops _____
EO/H _____ # of drops _____

Carrier Oils (CO) Used

CO _____ amount_____
CO _____ amount_____
CO _____ amount_____

Notes

_____
_____
_____
_____
_____
_____
_____
_____
_____
_____
_____
_____
_____

Preparation

_____
_____
_____
_____
_____
_____
_____
_____
_____
_____
_____
_____
_____
_____
_____
_____
_____

Blend Name

Love Factor
♡♡♡♡♡

How To Use

Ingredients ○

Purpose

Essential Oil (EO) and/or Hydrosol (H) Used _____
EO/H _____ # of drops _____ _____
EO/H _____ # of drops _____ _____
EO/H _____ # of drops _____ _____
EO/H _____ # of drops _____ _____
EO/H _____ # of drops _____ _____
EO/H _____ # of drops _____ _____

_____

Carrier Oils (CO) Used

_____

CO _____ amount_____ _____
CO _____ amount_____ _____
CO _____ amount_____ _____

Preparation

Notes ✏

_____ _____
_____ _____
_____ _____
_____ _____
_____ _____
_____ _____
_____ _____
_____ _____
_____ _____
_____ _____
_____ _____
_____ _____
_____ _____
_____ _____
_____ _____
_____ _____

Love Factor

♡ ♡ ♡ ♡ ♡

How To Use

Blend Name

Purpose

_____
_____
_____
_____
_____
_____
_____
_____
_____
_____

Ingredients ◊

Essential Oil (EO) and/or Hydrosol (H) Used

EO/H _____ # of drops _____
EO/H _____ # of drops _____
EO/H _____ # of drops _____
EO/H _____ # of drops _____
EO/H _____ # of drops _____
EO/H _____ # of drops _____

Carrier Oils (CO) Used

CO _____ amount_____
CO _____ amount_____
CO _____ amount_____

Notes 🖊

_____
_____
_____
_____
_____
_____
_____
_____
_____
_____
_____
_____
_____

Preparation

Blend Name

Love Factor
♡♡♡♡♡

How To Use

Ingredients 🜄

Essential Oil (EO) and/or Hydrosol (H) Used

EO/H _____ # of drops _____ _____
EO/H _____ # of drops _____ _____
EO/H _____ # of drops _____ _____
EO/H _____ # of drops _____ _____
EO/H _____ # of drops _____ _____
EO/H _____ # of drops _____ _____

Carrier Oils (CO) Used

CO _____ amount_____ _____
CO _____ amount_____ _____
CO _____ amount_____ _____

Purpose

_____
_____
_____
_____
_____
_____
_____
_____
_____
_____
_____

Preparation

_____
_____
_____
_____
_____
_____
_____
_____
_____
_____
_____
_____
_____
_____
_____

Notes ✏

_____
_____
_____
_____
_____
_____
_____
_____
_____
_____
_____
_____
_____

Love Factor

♡ ♡ ♡ ♡ ♡

How To Use

Blend Name

Purpose

_____
_____
_____
_____
_____
_____
_____
_____
_____
_____
_____

Ingredients ⬡

Essential Oil (EO) and/or Hydrosol (H) Used
EO/H _____ # of drops _____
EO/H _____ # of drops _____
EO/H _____ # of drops _____
EO/H _____ # of drops _____
EO/H _____ # of drops _____
EO/H _____ # of drops _____

Carrier Oils (CO) Used
CO _____ amount_____
CO _____ amount_____
CO _____ amount_____

Notes ✐

_____
_____
_____
_____
_____
_____
_____
_____
_____
_____
_____
_____
_____
_____

Preparation

_____
_____
_____
_____
_____
_____
_____
_____
_____
_____
_____
_____
_____
_____
_____
_____
_____

Blend Name

Love Factor
♡ ♡ ♡ ♡ ♡

How To Use

Ingredients 💧

Essential Oil (EO) and/or Hydrosol (H) Used _____

EO/H _____ # of drops _____ _____
EO/H _____ # of drops _____ _____
EO/H _____ # of drops _____ _____
EO/H _____ # of drops _____ _____
EO/H _____ # of drops _____ _____
EO/H _____ # of drops _____ _____

Purpose
_____

Carrier Oils (CO) Used
_____
CO _____ amount_____ _____
CO _____ amount_____ _____
CO _____ amount_____ _____

Preparation
_____
_____
_____
_____
_____
_____
_____
_____
_____
_____
_____
_____
_____
_____
_____

Notes ✏
_____
_____
_____
_____
_____
_____
_____
_____
_____
_____
_____
_____
_____
_____

Love Factor

♡ ♡ ♡ ♡ ♡

How To Use

Blend Name

Purpose

_____
_____
_____
_____
_____
_____
_____
_____
_____
_____
_____
_____

Ingredients ⬡

Essential Oil (EO) and/or Hydrosol (H) Used

EO/H _____ # of drops _____
EO/H _____ # of drops _____
EO/H _____ # of drops _____
EO/H _____ # of drops _____
EO/H _____ # of drops _____
EO/H _____ # of drops _____

Carrier Oils (CO) Used

CO _____ amount_____
CO _____ amount_____
CO _____ amount_____

Notes 🖉

_____
_____
_____
_____
_____
_____
_____
_____
_____
_____
_____
_____
_____
_____

Preparation

_____
_____
_____
_____
_____
_____
_____
_____
_____
_____
_____
_____
_____
_____
_____
_____
_____

Blend Name

Love Factor
♡♡♡♡♡

How To Use

Ingredients ⬦

Purpose

Essential Oil (EO) and/or Hydrosol (H) Used _____

EO/H _____ # of drops _____ _____
EO/H _____ # of drops _____ _____
EO/H _____ # of drops _____ _____
EO/H _____ # of drops _____ _____
EO/H _____ # of drops _____ _____
EO/H _____ # of drops _____ _____

_____

Carrier Oils (CO) Used

_____

CO _____ amount_____ _____
CO _____ amount_____ _____
CO _____ amount_____ _____

Preparation

Notes ✎

_____   _____
_____   _____
_____   _____
_____   _____
_____   _____
_____   _____
_____   _____
_____   _____
_____   _____
_____   _____
_____   _____
_____   _____
_____   _____
_____   _____
_____   _____
_____   _____

Love Factor

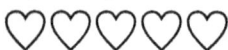

♡ ♡ ♡ ♡ ♡

How To Use

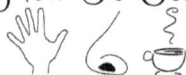

Blend Name

Purpose

_____
_____
_____
_____
_____
_____
_____
_____
_____
_____
_____

Ingredients 💧

Essential Oil (EO) and/or Hydrosol (H) Used

EO/H _____ # of drops _____
EO/H _____ # of drops _____
EO/H _____ # of drops _____
EO/H _____ # of drops _____
EO/H _____ # of drops _____
EO/H _____ # of drops _____

Carrier Oils (CO) Used

CO _____ amount_____
CO _____ amount_____
CO _____ amount_____

Notes ✏️

_____
_____
_____
_____
_____
_____
_____
_____
_____
_____
_____
_____
_____
_____
_____

Preparation

_____
_____
_____
_____
_____
_____
_____
_____
_____
_____
_____
_____
_____
_____
_____
_____
_____
_____
_____

Blend Name

Love Factor
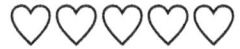

How To Use
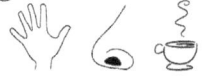

Ingredients ◯

Essential Oil (EO) and/or Hydrosol (H) Used _____

EO/H _____ # of drops _____ _____

EO/H _____ # of drops _____ _____

EO/H _____ # of drops _____ _____

EO/H _____ # of drops _____ _____

EO/H _____ # of drops _____ _____

EO/H _____ # of drops _____ _____

Carrier Oils (CO) Used

CO _____ amount_____ _____

CO _____ amount_____ _____

CO _____ amount_____ _____

Purpose

_____
_____
_____
_____
_____
_____
_____
_____
_____
_____

Preparation

_____
_____
_____
_____
_____
_____
_____
_____
_____
_____
_____
_____
_____
_____
_____
_____

Notes ✏

_____
_____
_____
_____
_____
_____
_____
_____
_____
_____
_____
_____
_____
_____

Love Factor

♡ ♡ ♡ ♡ ♡

How To Use

Blend Name

Purpose

_____
_____
_____
_____
_____
_____
_____
_____
_____
_____
_____

Ingredients ◊

Essential Oil (EO) and/or Hydrosol (H) Used

EO/H _____ # of drops _____
EO/H _____ # of drops _____
EO/H _____ # of drops _____
EO/H _____ # of drops _____
EO/H _____ # of drops _____
EO/H _____ # of drops _____

Carrier Oils (CO) Used

CO _____ amount_____
CO _____ amount_____
CO _____ amount_____

Notes ✏

_____
_____
_____
_____
_____
_____
_____
_____
_____
_____
_____
_____
_____
_____

Preparation

_____
_____
_____
_____
_____
_____
_____
_____
_____
_____
_____
_____
_____
_____
_____
_____

Blend Name

Love Factor
♡ ♡ ♡ ♡ ♡

How To Use

Ingredients ◌

Essential Oil (EO) and/or Hydrosol (H) Used

EO/H _____ # of drops _____
EO/H _____ # of drops _____
EO/H _____ # of drops _____
EO/H _____ # of drops _____
EO/H _____ # of drops _____
EO/H _____ # of drops _____

Carrier Oils (CO) Used

CO _____ amount_____
CO _____ amount_____
CO _____ amount_____

Purpose

_____
_____
_____
_____
_____
_____
_____
_____
_____
_____
_____

Preparation

_____
_____
_____
_____
_____
_____
_____
_____
_____
_____
_____
_____
_____
_____
_____
_____

Notes ✏

_____
_____
_____
_____
_____
_____
_____
_____
_____
_____
_____
_____
_____
_____

Love Factor
♡ ♡ ♡ ♡ ♡

How To Use

Blend Name

Purpose

_____
_____
_____
_____
_____
_____
_____
_____
_____
_____
_____
_____

Ingredients 🌢

Essential Oil (EO) and/or Hydrosol (H) Used

EO/H _____ # of drops _____
EO/H _____ # of drops _____
EO/H _____ # of drops _____
EO/H _____ # of drops _____
EO/H _____ # of drops _____
EO/H _____ # of drops _____

Carrier Oils (CO) Used

CO _____ amount_____
CO _____ amount_____
CO _____ amount_____

Notes ✏

_____
_____
_____
_____
_____
_____
_____
_____
_____
_____
_____
_____
_____
_____

Preparation

_____
_____
_____
_____
_____
_____
_____
_____
_____
_____
_____
_____
_____
_____
_____
_____
_____

Blend Name

Love Factor
♡ ♡ ♡ ♡ ♡

How To Use
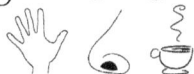

Ingredients ◌

Purpose _____

Essential Oil (EO) and/or Hydrosol (H) Used _____

EO/H _____ # of drops _____ _____
EO/H _____ # of drops _____ _____
EO/H _____ # of drops _____ _____
EO/H _____ # of drops _____ _____
EO/H _____ # of drops _____ _____
EO/H _____ # of drops _____ _____

_____

Carrier Oils (CO) Used _____

CO _____ amount_____ _____
CO _____ amount_____ _____
CO _____ amount_____ _____

Preparation

_____
_____
_____
_____
_____
_____
_____
_____
_____
_____
_____
_____
_____
_____
_____
_____

Notes ✏

_____
_____
_____
_____
_____
_____
_____
_____
_____
_____
_____
_____
_____
_____

Love Factor
♡ ♡ ♡ ♡ ♡

How To Use

Blend Name

Purpose

_____
_____
_____
_____
_____
_____
_____
_____
_____
_____
_____

Ingredients ⬭

Essential Oil (EO) and/or Hydrosol (H) Used
EO/H _____ # of drops _____
EO/H _____ # of drops _____
EO/H _____ # of drops _____
EO/H _____ # of drops _____
EO/H _____ # of drops _____
EO/H _____ # of drops _____

Carrier Oils (CO) Used
CO _____ amount_____
CO _____ amount_____
CO _____ amount_____

Notes ✏

_____
_____
_____
_____
_____
_____
_____
_____
_____
_____
_____
_____
_____
_____

Preparation

_____
_____
_____
_____
_____
_____
_____
_____
_____
_____
_____
_____
_____
_____
_____
_____
_____

Blend Name

Love Factor
♡ ♡ ♡ ♡ ♡

How To Use

Ingredients ⬡

Essential Oil (EO) and/or Hydrosol (H) Used

EO/H _____ # of drops _____
EO/H _____ # of drops _____
EO/H _____ # of drops _____
EO/H _____ # of drops _____
EO/H _____ # of drops _____
EO/H _____ # of drops _____

Carrier Oils (CO) Used

CO _____ amount_____
CO _____ amount_____
CO _____ amount_____

Purpose
_____
_____
_____
_____
_____
_____
_____
_____
_____
_____

Preparation
_____
_____
_____
_____
_____
_____
_____
_____
_____
_____
_____
_____
_____
_____
_____

Notes ✏
_____
_____
_____
_____
_____
_____
_____
_____
_____
_____
_____
_____

Love Factor

♡ ♡ ♡ ♡ ♡

How To Use

Blend Name

Purpose

_____
_____
_____
_____
_____
_____
_____
_____
_____
_____
_____

Ingredients ◊

Essential Oil (EO) and/or Hydrosol (H) Used

EO/H _____ # of drops _____
EO/H _____ # of drops _____
EO/H _____ # of drops _____
EO/H _____ # of drops _____
EO/H _____ # of drops _____
EO/H _____ # of drops _____

Carrier Oils (CO) Used

CO _____ amount_____
CO _____ amount_____
CO _____ amount_____

Notes ✏

_____
_____
_____
_____
_____
_____
_____
_____
_____
_____
_____
_____
_____

Preparation

_____
_____
_____
_____
_____
_____
_____
_____
_____
_____
_____
_____
_____
_____
_____
_____
_____

Blend Name

Love Factor
♡♡♡♡♡

How To Use

Ingredients ◯

Essential Oil (EO) and/or Hydrosol (H) Used _____

EO/H _____ # of drops _____ _____

EO/H _____ # of drops _____ _____

EO/H _____ # of drops _____ _____

EO/H _____ # of drops _____ _____

EO/H _____ # of drops _____ _____

EO/H _____ # of drops _____

Purpose

_____

_____

Carrier Oils (CO) Used

CO _____ amount_____ _____

CO _____ amount_____ _____

CO _____ amount_____ _____

Preparation

_____

_____

_____

_____

_____

_____

_____

_____

_____

_____

_____

_____

_____

_____

_____

_____

Notes ✏

_____

_____

_____

_____

_____

_____

_____

_____

_____

_____

_____

_____

_____

_____

Love Factor

♡ ♡ ♡ ♡ ♡

How To Use

Blend Name

Purpose

_____
_____
_____
_____
_____
_____
_____
_____
_____
_____
_____

Ingredients 💧

Essential Oil (EO) and/or Hydrosol (H) Used
EO/H _____ # of drops _____
EO/H _____ # of drops _____
EO/H _____ # of drops _____
EO/H _____ # of drops _____
EO/H _____ # of drops _____
EO/H _____ # of drops _____

Carrier Oils (CO) Used
CO _____ amount_____
CO _____ amount_____
CO _____ amount_____

Notes ✏

_____
_____
_____
_____
_____
_____
_____
_____
_____
_____
_____
_____
_____
_____

Preparation

_____
_____
_____
_____
_____
_____
_____
_____
_____
_____
_____
_____
_____
_____
_____
_____
_____

Blend Name

Love Factor

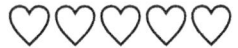

How To Use

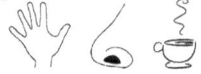

Ingredients 💧

Essential Oil (EO) and/or Hydrosol (H) Used _____

Purpose

EO/H _____ # of drops _____ _____
EO/H _____ # of drops _____ _____
EO/H _____ # of drops _____ _____
EO/H _____ # of drops _____ _____
EO/H _____ # of drops _____ _____
EO/H _____ # of drops _____ _____

_____

Carrier Oils (CO) Used
CO _____ amount_____ _____
CO _____ amount_____ _____
CO _____ amount_____ _____

Preparation

_____

Notes ✏️

_____
_____
_____
_____
_____
_____
_____
_____
_____
_____
_____
_____
_____
_____
_____

Love Factor

♡ ♡ ♡ ♡ ♡

How To Use

Blend Name

Purpose

_____
_____
_____
_____
_____
_____
_____
_____
_____
_____
_____

Ingredients ⬦

Essential Oil (EO) and/or Hydrosol (H) Used

EO/H _____ # of drops _____
EO/H _____ # of drops _____
EO/H _____ # of drops _____
EO/H _____ # of drops _____
EO/H _____ # of drops _____
EO/H _____ # of drops _____

Carrier Oils (CO) Used

CO _____ amount_____
CO _____ amount_____
CO _____ amount_____

Notes ✏

_____
_____
_____
_____
_____
_____
_____
_____
_____
_____
_____
_____
_____
_____

Preparation

_____
_____
_____
_____
_____
_____
_____
_____
_____
_____
_____
_____
_____
_____
_____
_____
_____
_____

Blend Name

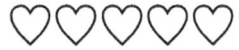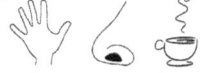
Ingredients 💧

Essential Oil (EO) and/or Hydrosol (H) Used

EO/H _____ # of drops _____
EO/H _____ # of drops _____
EO/H _____ # of drops _____
EO/H _____ # of drops _____
EO/H _____ # of drops _____
EO/H _____ # of drops _____

Carrier Oils (CO) Used

CO _____ amount_____
CO _____ amount_____
CO _____ amount_____

Purpose

_____
_____
_____
_____
_____
_____
_____
_____
_____
_____

Preparation

_____
_____
_____
_____
_____
_____
_____
_____
_____
_____
_____
_____
_____
_____
_____
_____

Notes ✏️

_____
_____
_____
_____
_____
_____
_____
_____
_____
_____
_____
_____
_____
_____

123

Love Factor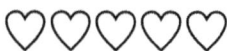

♡ ♡ ♡ ♡ ♡

How To Use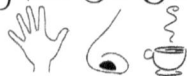

Blend Name

Purpose

_____
_____
_____
_____
_____
_____
_____
_____
_____
_____

Ingredients

Essential Oil (EO) and/or Hydrosol (H) Used

EO/H _____ # of drops _____
EO/H _____ # of drops _____
EO/H _____ # of drops _____
EO/H _____ # of drops _____
EO/H _____ # of drops _____
EO/H _____ # of drops _____

Carrier Oils (CO) Used

CO _____ amount_____
CO _____ amount_____
CO _____ amount_____

Notes 🖉

_____
_____
_____
_____
_____
_____
_____
_____
_____
_____
_____
_____
_____
_____

Preparation

_____
_____
_____
_____
_____
_____
_____
_____
_____
_____
_____
_____
_____
_____
_____
_____
_____

Blend Name

Love Factor
♡♡♡♡♡

How To Use
✋ 👁 ☕

Ingredients ○

Essential Oil (EO) and/or Hydrosol (H) Used

EO/H _____ # of drops _____
EO/H _____ # of drops _____
EO/H _____ # of drops _____
EO/H _____ # of drops _____
EO/H _____ # of drops _____
EO/H _____ # of drops _____

Carrier Oils (CO) Used

CO _____ amount_____
CO _____ amount_____
CO _____ amount_____

Purpose

_____
_____
_____
_____
_____
_____
_____
_____
_____
_____
_____
_____

Preparation

_____
_____
_____
_____
_____
_____
_____
_____
_____
_____
_____
_____
_____
_____
_____
_____
_____

Notes ✏

_____
_____
_____
_____
_____
_____
_____
_____
_____
_____
_____
_____
_____
_____

125

Love Factor

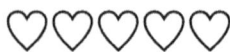

How To Use

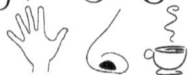

Blend Name

Purpose

_____
_____
_____
_____
_____
_____
_____
_____
_____
_____
_____

Ingredients ⬦

Essential Oil (EO) and/or Hydrosol (H) Used
EO/H _____ # of drops _____
EO/H _____ # of drops _____
EO/H _____ # of drops _____
EO/H _____ # of drops _____
EO/H _____ # of drops _____
EO/H _____ # of drops _____

Carrier Oils (CO) Used
CO _____ amount_____
CO _____ amount_____
CO _____ amount_____

Notes ✎

_____
_____
_____
_____
_____
_____
_____
_____
_____
_____
_____
_____
_____
_____

Preparation

_____
_____
_____
_____
_____
_____
_____
_____
_____
_____
_____
_____
_____
_____
_____
_____
_____

Blend Name

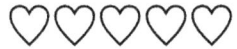

How To Use

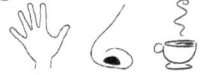

Ingredients △

Purpose

Essential Oil (EO) and/or Hydrosol (H) Used _____

EO/H _____ # of drops _____ _____

EO/H _____ # of drops _____ _____

EO/H _____ # of drops _____ _____

EO/H _____ # of drops _____ _____

EO/H _____ # of drops _____ _____

EO/H _____ # of drops _____ _____

Carrier Oils (CO) Used

CO _____ amount_____ _____

CO _____ amount_____ _____

CO _____ amount_____ _____

Preparation

Notes ✏

_____ _____

_____ _____

_____ _____

_____ _____

_____ _____

_____ _____

_____ _____

_____ _____

_____ _____

_____ _____

_____ _____

_____ _____

_____ _____

_____ _____

_____

Love Factor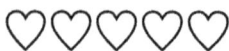

Blend Name

How To Use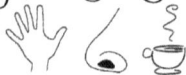

Purpose

_____
_____
_____
_____
_____
_____
_____
_____
_____
_____
_____
_____

Ingredients

Essential Oil (EO) and/or Hydrosol (H) Used
EO/H _____ # of drops _____
EO/H _____ # of drops _____
EO/H _____ # of drops _____
EO/H _____ # of drops _____
EO/H _____ # of drops _____
EO/H _____ # of drops _____

Carrier Oils (CO) Used
CO _____ amount_____
CO _____ amount_____
CO _____ amount_____

Notes

_____
_____
_____
_____
_____
_____
_____
_____
_____
_____
_____
_____
_____
_____
_____

Preparation

_____
_____
_____
_____
_____
_____
_____
_____
_____
_____
_____
_____
_____
_____
_____
_____
_____
_____

Blend Name

Love Factor
♡ ♡ ♡ ♡ ♡

How To Use

Ingredients 🌢

Essential Oil (EO) and/or Hydrosol (H) Used

EO/H _____ # of drops _____
EO/H _____ # of drops _____
EO/H _____ # of drops _____
EO/H _____ # of drops _____
EO/H _____ # of drops _____
EO/H _____ # of drops _____

Carrier Oils (CO) Used

CO _____ amount_____
CO _____ amount_____
CO _____ amount_____

Preparation

_____
_____
_____
_____
_____
_____
_____
_____
_____
_____
_____
_____
_____
_____
_____
_____

Purpose

_____
_____
_____
_____
_____
_____
_____
_____
_____
_____
_____
_____

Notes ✏

_____
_____
_____
_____
_____
_____
_____
_____
_____
_____
_____
_____
_____

129

Love Factor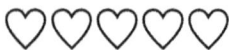
♡ ♡ ♡ ♡ ♡

How To Use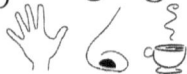

Blend Name

Purpose

_____
_____
_____
_____
_____
_____
_____
_____
_____
_____
_____

Ingredients ◊

Essential Oil (EO) and/or Hydrosol (H) Used
EO/H _____ # of drops _____
EO/H _____ # of drops _____
EO/H _____ # of drops _____
EO/H _____ # of drops _____
EO/H _____ # of drops _____
EO/H _____ # of drops _____

Carrier Oils (CO) Used
CO _____ amount_____
CO _____ amount_____
CO _____ amount_____

Notes 🖉

Preparation

Blend Name

Love Factor
♡♡♡♡♡

How To Use

Ingredients ○

Purpose

Essential Oil (EO) and/or Hydrosol (H) Used _____
EO/H _____ # of drops _____ _____
EO/H _____ # of drops _____ _____
EO/H _____ # of drops _____ _____
EO/H _____ # of drops _____ _____
EO/H _____ # of drops _____ _____
EO/H _____ # of drops _____ _____

_____

Carrier Oils (CO) Used
CO _____ amount_____ _____
CO _____ amount_____ _____
CO _____ amount_____ _____

Preparation

Notes ✏

_____ _____
_____ _____
_____ _____
_____ _____
_____ _____
_____ _____
_____ _____
_____ _____
_____ _____
_____ _____
_____ _____
_____ _____
_____ _____
_____ _____
_____ _____
_____

Love Factor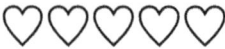

Blend Name

How To Use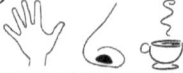

Purpose

_____
_____
_____
_____
_____
_____
_____
_____
_____
_____

Ingredients ○

Essential Oil (EO) and/or Hydrosol (H) Used

EO/H _____ # of drops _____
EO/H _____ # of drops _____
EO/H _____ # of drops _____
EO/H _____ # of drops _____
EO/H _____ # of drops _____
EO/H _____ # of drops _____

Carrier Oils (CO) Used

CO _____ amount_____
CO _____ amount_____
CO _____ amount_____

Notes 🖉

_____
_____
_____
_____
_____
_____
_____
_____
_____
_____
_____
_____
_____
_____

Preparation

_____
_____
_____
_____
_____
_____
_____
_____
_____
_____
_____
_____
_____
_____
_____
_____

Blend Name

Love Factor

♡ ♡ ♡ ♡ ♡

How To Use

Ingredients ◊

Essential Oil (EO) and/or Hydrosol (H) Used

Purpose

_____

EO/H _____ # of drops _____ _____

EO/H _____ # of drops _____ _____

EO/H _____ # of drops _____ _____

EO/H _____ # of drops _____ _____

EO/H _____ # of drops _____ _____

EO/H _____ # of drops _____ _____

_____

Carrier Oils (CO) Used

_____

CO _____ amount_____ _____

CO _____ amount_____ _____

CO _____ amount_____ _____

Preparation

Notes ✏

_____ _____

_____ _____

_____ _____

_____ _____

_____ _____

_____ _____

_____ _____

_____ _____

_____ _____

_____ _____

_____ _____

_____ _____

_____ _____

_____ _____

_____ _____

_____ _____

_____ _____

Love Factor
♡ ♡ ♡ ♡ ♡

How To Use

Blend Name

Purpose

_____
_____
_____
_____
_____
_____
_____
_____
_____
_____
_____
_____

Ingredients

Essential Oil (EO) and/or Hydrosol (H) Used

EO/H _____ # of drops _____
EO/H _____ # of drops _____
EO/H _____ # of drops _____
EO/H _____ # of drops _____
EO/H _____ # of drops _____
EO/H _____ # of drops _____

Carrier Oils (CO) Used

CO _____ amount_____
CO _____ amount_____
CO _____ amount_____

Notes

_____
_____
_____
_____
_____
_____
_____
_____
_____
_____
_____
_____
_____
_____
_____

Preparation

_____
_____
_____
_____
_____
_____
_____
_____
_____
_____
_____
_____
_____
_____
_____
_____
_____
_____

Blend Name

Love Factor
♡ ♡ ♡ ♡ ♡

How To Use

Ingredients ⬭

Purpose

Essential Oil (EO) and/or Hydrosol (H) Used _____
EO/H _____ # of drops _____ _____
EO/H _____ # of drops _____ _____
EO/H _____ # of drops _____ _____
EO/H _____ # of drops _____ _____
EO/H _____ # of drops _____ _____
EO/H _____ # of drops _____ _____

_____

Carrier Oils (CO) Used _____
CO _____ amount_____ _____
CO _____ amount_____ _____
CO _____ amount_____ _____

Preparation

Notes ✎

_____ _____
_____ _____
_____ _____
_____ _____
_____ _____
_____ _____
_____ _____
_____ _____
_____ _____
_____ _____
_____ _____
_____ _____
_____ _____
_____ _____
_____ _____

_____

Love Factor

♡ ♡ ♡ ♡ ♡

How To Use

Blend Name

Purpose

_____
_____
_____
_____
_____
_____
_____
_____
_____
_____
_____

Ingredients

Essential Oil (EO) and/or **Hydrosol (H) Used**

EO/H _____ # of drops _____
EO/H _____ # of drops _____
EO/H _____ # of drops _____
EO/H _____ # of drops _____
EO/H _____ # of drops _____
EO/H _____ # of drops _____

Carrier Oils (CO) Used

CO _____ amount_____
CO _____ amount_____
CO _____ amount_____

Notes

_____
_____
_____
_____
_____
_____
_____
_____
_____
_____
_____
_____
_____
_____
_____

Preparation

_____
_____
_____
_____
_____
_____
_____
_____
_____
_____
_____
_____
_____
_____
_____
_____
_____

Blend Name

Love Factor

♡♡♡♡♡

How To Use

Ingredients ⬡

Purpose

Essential Oil (EO) and/or Hydrosol (H) Used _____

EO/H _____ # of drops _____ _____

EO/H _____ # of drops _____ _____

EO/H _____ # of drops _____ _____

EO/H _____ # of drops _____ _____

EO/H _____ # of drops _____ _____

EO/H _____ # of drops _____ _____

_____

Carrier Oils (CO) Used

_____

CO _____ amount_____ _____

CO _____ amount_____ _____

CO _____ amount_____ _____

Preparation

Notes ✏

_____ _____

_____ _____

_____ _____

_____ _____

_____ _____

_____ _____

_____ _____

_____ _____

_____ _____

_____ _____

_____ _____

_____ _____

_____ _____

_____ _____

137

Love Factor

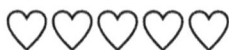

How To Use

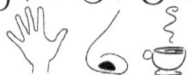

Blend Name

Purpose

_____
_____
_____
_____
_____
_____
_____
_____
_____
_____
_____

Ingredients

Essential Oil (EO) and/or Hydrosol (H) Used

EO/H _____ # of drops _____
EO/H _____ # of drops _____
EO/H _____ # of drops _____
EO/H _____ # of drops _____
EO/H _____ # of drops _____
EO/H _____ # of drops _____

Carrier Oils (CO) Used

CO _____ amount_____
CO _____ amount_____
CO _____ amount_____

Notes

_____
_____
_____
_____
_____
_____
_____
_____
_____
_____
_____
_____
_____
_____

Preparation

_____
_____
_____
_____
_____
_____
_____
_____
_____
_____
_____
_____
_____
_____
_____
_____

Blend Name

Love Factor
♡♡♡♡♡

How To Use

Ingredients 💧

Purpose _____

Essential Oil (EO) and/or Hydrosol (H) Used

EO/H _____ # of drops _____ _____
EO/H _____ # of drops _____ _____
EO/H _____ # of drops _____ _____
EO/H _____ # of drops _____ _____
EO/H _____ # of drops _____ _____
EO/H _____ # of drops _____ _____

_____

Carrier Oils (CO) Used

_____

CO _____ amount_____ _____
CO _____ amount_____ _____
CO _____ amount_____ _____

Preparation

Notes ✏

_____ _____
_____ _____
_____ _____
_____ _____
_____ _____
_____ _____
_____ _____
_____ _____
_____ _____
_____ _____
_____ _____
_____ _____
_____ _____
_____ _____
_____ _____
_____ _____
_____ _____

139

Love Factor
♡ ♡ ♡ ♡ ♡

How To Use

Blend Name

Purpose

_____
_____
_____
_____
_____
_____
_____
_____
_____
_____
_____

Ingredients ◇

Essential Oil (EO) and/or Hydrosol (H) Used
EO/H _____ # of drops _____
EO/H _____ # of drops _____
EO/H _____ # of drops _____
EO/H _____ # of drops _____
EO/H _____ # of drops _____
EO/H _____ # of drops _____

Carrier Oils (CO) Used
CO _____ amount_____
CO _____ amount_____
CO _____ amount_____

Notes ✏

_____
_____
_____
_____
_____
_____
_____
_____
_____
_____
_____
_____
_____

140

Preparation

_____
_____
_____
_____
_____
_____
_____
_____
_____
_____
_____
_____
_____
_____
_____
_____

Blend Name

Love Factor
♡ ♡ ♡ ♡ ♡

How To Use

Ingredients 🜄

Essential Oil (EO) and/or Hydrosol (H) Used

Purpose

_____

EO/H _____ # of drops _____ _____

EO/H _____ # of drops _____ _____

EO/H _____ # of drops _____ _____

EO/H _____ # of drops _____ _____

EO/H _____ # of drops _____ _____

EO/H _____ # of drops _____ _____

_____

Carrier Oils (CO) Used _____

CO _____ amount_____ _____

CO _____ amount_____ _____

CO _____ amount_____ _____

Preparation

Notes 🖉

_____ _____
_____ _____
_____ _____
_____ _____
_____ _____
_____ _____
_____ _____
_____ _____
_____ _____
_____ _____
_____ _____
_____ _____
_____ _____
_____ _____
_____ _____

141

Love Factor

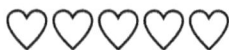

♡ ♡ ♡ ♡ ♡

How To Use

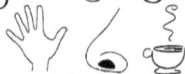

Blend Name

Purpose

_____
_____
_____
_____
_____
_____
_____
_____
_____
_____
_____

Ingredients ⬡

Essential Oil (EO) and/or **Hydrosol (H) Used**

EO/H _____ # of drops _____
EO/H _____ # of drops _____
EO/H _____ # of drops _____
EO/H _____ # of drops _____
EO/H _____ # of drops _____
EO/H _____ # of drops _____

Carrier Oils (CO) Used

CO _____ amount_____
CO _____ amount_____
CO _____ amount_____

Notes ✏

_____
_____
_____
_____
_____
_____
_____
_____
_____
_____
_____
_____
_____
_____

Preparation

_____
_____
_____
_____
_____
_____
_____
_____
_____
_____
_____
_____
_____
_____
_____
_____
_____
_____

Blend Name

Love Factor
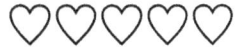

How To Use
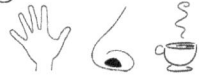

Ingredients

Essential Oil (EO) and/or Hydrosol (H) Used _____

EO/H _____ # of drops _____ _____
EO/H _____ # of drops _____ _____
EO/H _____ # of drops _____ _____
EO/H _____ # of drops _____ _____
EO/H _____ # of drops _____ _____
EO/H _____ # of drops _____ _____

Purpose
_____
_____
_____

Carrier Oils (CO) Used
_____

CO _____ amount_____ _____
CO _____ amount_____ _____
CO _____ amount_____ _____

Preparation

_____
_____
_____
_____
_____
_____
_____
_____
_____
_____
_____
_____
_____
_____
_____

Notes

_____
_____
_____
_____
_____
_____
_____
_____
_____
_____
_____
_____

Love Factor

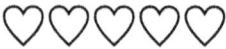
♡ ♡ ♡ ♡ ♡

How To Use

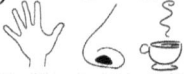

Blend Name

Purpose

_____
_____
_____
_____
_____
_____
_____
_____
_____
_____
_____

Ingredients ⬭

Essential Oil (EO) and/or Hydrosol (H) Used

EO/H _____ # of drops _____
EO/H _____ # of drops _____
EO/H _____ # of drops _____
EO/H _____ # of drops _____
EO/H _____ # of drops _____
EO/H _____ # of drops _____

Carrier Oils (CO) Used

CO _____ amount_____
CO _____ amount_____
CO _____ amount_____

Notes ✏

_____
_____
_____
_____
_____
_____
_____
_____
_____
_____
_____
_____
_____
_____

Preparation

_____
_____
_____
_____
_____
_____
_____
_____
_____
_____
_____
_____
_____
_____
_____
_____
_____

Blend Name

Love Factor
♡ ♡ ♡ ♡ ♡

How To Use
🖐 👃 ☕

Ingredients 💧

Essential Oil (EO) and/or Hydrosol (H) Used

EO/H _____ # of drops _____
EO/H _____ # of drops _____
EO/H _____ # of drops _____
EO/H _____ # of drops _____
EO/H _____ # of drops _____
EO/H _____ # of drops _____

Carrier Oils (CO) Used

CO _____ amount_____
CO _____ amount_____
CO _____ amount_____

Purpose
_____
_____
_____
_____
_____
_____
_____
_____
_____
_____
_____

Preparation
_____
_____
_____
_____
_____
_____
_____
_____
_____
_____
_____
_____
_____
_____
_____
_____

Notes ✏
_____
_____
_____
_____
_____
_____
_____
_____
_____
_____
_____
_____
_____
_____

Love Factor

♡ ♡ ♡ ♡ ♡

How To Use

Blend Name

Purpose

_____
_____
_____
_____
_____
_____
_____
_____
_____
_____
_____

Ingredients ◌

Essential Oil (EO) and/or Hydrosol (H) Used

EO/H _____ # of drops _____
EO/H _____ # of drops _____
EO/H _____ # of drops _____
EO/H _____ # of drops _____
EO/H _____ # of drops _____
EO/H _____ # of drops _____

Carrier Oils (CO) Used

CO _____ amount_____
CO _____ amount_____
CO _____ amount_____

Notes 🖉

Preparation

Blend Name

Love Factor
♡♡♡♡♡

How To Use
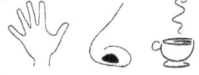

Ingredients ◇

Essential Oil (EO) and/or Hydrosol (H) Used _____

Purpose

EO/H _____ # of drops _____ _____
EO/H _____ # of drops _____ _____
EO/H _____ # of drops _____ _____
EO/H _____ # of drops _____ _____
EO/H _____ # of drops _____ _____
EO/H _____ # of drops _____ _____

_____

Carrier Oils (CO) Used

_____

CO _____ amount_____ _____
CO _____ amount_____ _____
CO _____ amount_____ _____

Preparation

Notes ✏

_____ _____
_____ _____
_____ _____
_____ _____
_____ _____
_____ _____
_____ _____
_____ _____
_____ _____
_____ _____
_____ _____
_____ _____
_____ _____
_____ _____
_____ _____
_____ _____

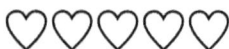
Love Factor

♡ ♡ ♡ ♡ ♡

How To Use
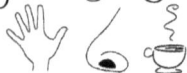

Blend Name

Purpose

_____
_____
_____
_____
_____
_____
_____
_____
_____
_____
_____

Ingredients ⬳

Essential Oil (EO) and/or **Hydrosol (H) Used**

EO/H _____ # of drops _____
EO/H _____ # of drops _____
EO/H _____ # of drops _____
EO/H _____ # of drops _____
EO/H _____ # of drops _____
EO/H _____ # of drops _____

Carrier Oils (CO) Used

CO _____ amount_____
CO _____ amount_____
CO _____ amount_____

Notes ✐

_____
_____
_____
_____
_____
_____
_____
_____
_____
_____
_____
_____
_____
_____

Preparation

_____
_____
_____
_____
_____
_____
_____
_____
_____
_____
_____
_____
_____
_____
_____
_____
_____
_____

Blend Name

Love Factor
♡ ♡ ♡ ♡ ♡

How To Use

Ingredients ⬭

Essential Oil (EO) and/or Hydrosol (H) Used _____

EO/H _____ # of drops _____ _____
EO/H _____ # of drops _____ _____
EO/H _____ # of drops _____ _____
EO/H _____ # of drops _____ _____
EO/H _____ # of drops _____ _____
EO/H _____ # of drops _____ _____

Purpose

_____

Carrier Oils (CO) Used

CO _____ amount_____ _____
CO _____ amount_____ _____
CO _____ amount_____ _____

Preparation

_____
_____
_____
_____
_____
_____
_____
_____
_____
_____
_____
_____
_____
_____

Notes ✏

_____
_____
_____
_____
_____
_____
_____
_____
_____
_____
_____
_____
_____

Love Factor
♡ ♡ ♡ ♡ ♡

Blend Name

How To Use

Purpose

_____
_____
_____
_____
_____
_____
_____
_____
_____
_____
_____
_____

Ingredients ⬭

Essential Oil (EO) and/or Hydrosol (H) Used
EO/H _____ # of drops _____
EO/H _____ # of drops _____
EO/H _____ # of drops _____
EO/H _____ # of drops _____
EO/H _____ # of drops _____
EO/H _____ # of drops _____

Carrier Oils (CO) Used
CO _____ amount_____
CO _____ amount_____
CO _____ amount_____

Notes ✏

_____
_____
_____
_____
_____
_____
_____
_____
_____
_____
_____
_____
_____
_____

Preparation

_____
_____
_____
_____
_____
_____
_____
_____
_____
_____
_____
_____
_____
_____
_____
_____

Blend Name

Love Factor
♡♡♡♡♡

How To Use
🖐 👃 ☕

Ingredients ◌

Essential Oil (EO) and/or Hydrosol (H) Used

EO/H _____ # of drops _____
EO/H _____ # of drops _____
EO/H _____ # of drops _____
EO/H _____ # of drops _____
EO/H _____ # of drops _____
EO/H _____ # of drops _____

Carrier Oils (CO) Used

CO _____ amount_____
CO _____ amount_____
CO _____ amount_____

Purpose

_____
_____
_____
_____
_____
_____
_____
_____
_____
_____
_____

Preparation

_____
_____
_____
_____
_____
_____
_____
_____
_____
_____
_____
_____
_____
_____
_____
_____

Notes ✏

_____
_____
_____
_____
_____
_____
_____
_____
_____
_____
_____
_____
_____
_____

Love Factor

♡ ♡ ♡ ♡ ♡

How To Use

Blend Name

Purpose

_____
_____
_____
_____
_____
_____
_____
_____
_____
_____
_____

Ingredients 💧

Essential Oil (EO) and/or Hydrosol (H) Used
EO/H _____ # of drops _____
EO/H _____ # of drops _____
EO/H _____ # of drops _____
EO/H _____ # of drops _____
EO/H _____ # of drops _____
EO/H _____ # of drops _____

Carrier Oils (CO) Used
CO _____ amount _____
CO _____ amount _____
CO _____ amount _____

Notes ✏️

_____
_____
_____
_____
_____
_____
_____
_____
_____
_____
_____
_____
_____
_____
_____
152

Preparation

_____
_____
_____
_____
_____
_____
_____
_____
_____
_____
_____
_____
_____
_____
_____
_____
_____

Blend Name

Love Factor
♡ ♡ ♡ ♡ ♡

How To Use

Ingredients ◌

Essential Oil (EO) and/or Hydrosol (H) Used

EO/H _____ # of drops _____

EO/H _____ # of drops _____

EO/H _____ # of drops _____

EO/H _____ # of drops _____

EO/H _____ # of drops _____

EO/H _____ # of drops _____

Carrier Oils (CO) Used

CO _____ amount_____

CO _____ amount_____

CO _____ amount_____

Purpose
_____
_____
_____
_____
_____
_____
_____
_____
_____
_____
_____

Preparation
_____
_____
_____
_____
_____
_____
_____
_____
_____
_____
_____
_____
_____
_____
_____

Notes ✏
_____
_____
_____
_____
_____
_____
_____
_____
_____
_____
_____
_____

153

Love Factor

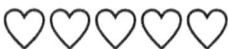

♡ ♡ ♡ ♡ ♡

How To Use

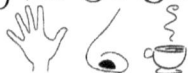

Blend Name

Purpose

_____
_____
_____
_____
_____
_____
_____
_____
_____
_____
_____

Ingredients 💧

Essential Oil (EO) and/or Hydrosol (H) Used

EO/H _____ # of drops _____
EO/H _____ # of drops _____
EO/H _____ # of drops _____
EO/H _____ # of drops _____
EO/H _____ # of drops _____
EO/H _____ # of drops _____

Carrier Oils (CO) Used

CO _____ amount_____
CO _____ amount_____
CO _____ amount_____

Notes ✏

_____
_____
_____
_____
_____
_____
_____
_____
_____
_____
_____
_____
_____
_____
_____

154

Preparation

_____
_____
_____
_____
_____
_____
_____
_____
_____
_____
_____
_____
_____
_____
_____
_____
_____
_____

Blend Name

Love Factor
♡♡♡♡♡

How To Use

Ingredients ⬭

Essential Oil (EO) and/or Hydrosol (H) Used

EO/H _____ # of drops _____

EO/H _____ # of drops _____

EO/H _____ # of drops _____

EO/H _____ # of drops _____

EO/H _____ # of drops _____

EO/H _____ # of drops _____

Carrier Oils (CO) Used

CO _____ amount_____

CO _____ amount_____

CO _____ amount_____

Purpose

_____
_____
_____
_____
_____
_____
_____
_____
_____
_____
_____

Preparation

_____
_____
_____
_____
_____
_____
_____
_____
_____
_____
_____
_____
_____
_____
_____

Notes ✏

_____
_____
_____
_____
_____
_____
_____
_____
_____
_____
_____
_____
_____
_____

Love Factor

♡ ♡ ♡ ♡ ♡

How To Use

Blend Name

Purpose

_____
_____
_____
_____
_____
_____
_____
_____
_____
_____

Ingredients ◌

Essential Oil (EO) and/or Hydrosol (H) Used

EO/H _____ # of drops _____
EO/H _____ # of drops _____
EO/H _____ # of drops _____
EO/H _____ # of drops _____
EO/H _____ # of drops _____
EO/H _____ # of drops _____

Carrier Oils (CO) Used

CO _____ amount_____
CO _____ amount_____
CO _____ amount_____

Notes ✎

_____
_____
_____
_____
_____
_____
_____
_____
_____
_____
_____
_____
_____
_____

156

Preparation

_____
_____
_____
_____
_____
_____
_____
_____
_____
_____
_____
_____
_____
_____
_____
_____

Blend Name

Love Factor
♡ ♡ ♡ ♡ ♡

How To Use

🖐 👃 ☕

Ingredients 💧

Purpose

Essential Oil (EO) and/or Hydrosol (H) Used _____
EO/H _____ # of drops _____ _____
EO/H _____ # of drops _____ _____
EO/H _____ # of drops _____ _____
EO/H _____ # of drops _____ _____
EO/H _____ # of drops _____ _____
EO/H _____ # of drops _____ _____

_____

Carrier Oils (CO) Used
CO _____ amount_____ _____
CO _____ amount_____ _____
CO _____ amount_____ _____

Preparation

Notes ✏

_____ _____
_____ _____
_____ _____
_____ _____
_____ _____
_____ _____
_____ _____
_____ _____
_____ _____
_____ _____
_____ _____
_____ _____
_____ _____
_____ _____
_____ _____
_____ _____
_____ _____

Love Factor

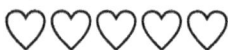

How To Use

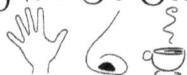

Blend Name

Purpose

_____
_____
_____
_____
_____
_____
_____
_____
_____
_____
_____

Ingredients 💧

Essential Oil (EO) and/or Hydrosol (H) Used

EO/H _____ # of drops _____
EO/H _____ # of drops _____
EO/H _____ # of drops _____
EO/H _____ # of drops _____
EO/H _____ # of drops _____
EO/H _____ # of drops _____

Carrier Oils (CO) Used

CO _____ amount_____
CO _____ amount_____
CO _____ amount_____

Notes 🖉

_____
_____
_____
_____
_____
_____
_____
_____
_____
_____
_____
_____
_____
_____

Preparation

_____
_____
_____
_____
_____
_____
_____
_____
_____
_____
_____
_____
_____
_____
_____
_____
_____
_____

Blend Name

Love Factor
♡♡♡♡♡

How To Use

Ingredients ⬳

Purpose

Essential Oil (EO) and/or Hydrosol (H) Used _____
EO/H _____ # of drops _____ _____
EO/H _____ # of drops _____ _____
EO/H _____ # of drops _____ _____
EO/H _____ # of drops _____ _____
EO/H _____ # of drops _____ _____
EO/H _____ # of drops _____ _____

_____

Carrier Oils (CO) Used
CO _____ amount_____ _____
CO _____ amount_____ _____
CO _____ amount_____ _____

Preparation

Notes ✎

_____ _____
_____ _____
_____ _____
_____ _____
_____ _____
_____ _____
_____ _____
_____ _____
_____ _____
_____ _____
_____ _____
_____ _____
_____ _____
_____ _____
_____ _____
_____ _____
_____ 159
_____

Love Factor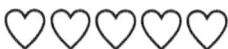
♡ ♡ ♡ ♡ ♡

How To Use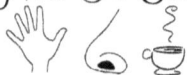

Blend Name

Purpose

_____
_____
_____
_____
_____
_____
_____
_____
_____
_____
_____

Ingredients ⬭

Essential Oil (EO) and/or Hydrosol (H) Used
EO/H _____ # of drops _____
EO/H _____ # of drops _____
EO/H _____ # of drops _____
EO/H _____ # of drops _____
EO/H _____ # of drops _____
EO/H _____ # of drops _____

Carrier Oils (CO) Used
CO _____ amount_____
CO _____ amount_____
CO _____ amount_____

Notes ✏

_____
_____
_____
_____
_____
_____
_____
_____
_____
_____
_____
_____
_____
_____
160

Preparation

_____
_____
_____
_____
_____
_____
_____
_____
_____
_____
_____
_____
_____
_____
_____
_____
_____
_____

Notes

Notes

Notes

Notes

Notes

_____
_____
_____
_____
_____
_____
_____
_____
_____
_____
_____
_____
_____
_____
_____
_____
_____
_____
_____
_____
_____
_____
_____
_____
_____
_____
_____
_____
_____
_____

Notes

Notes

Notes

Notes